Doc, I Want My Brain Back

My HBOT Miracle

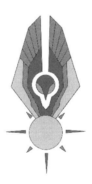

Dan Greathouse

DEDICATION

First, I'd like to dedicate this book to my parents, Betty and Jack Greathouse, and to my brother, Ross Greathouse. They refused to give up during my darkest hours, and I never take for granted what they did for me.

I also dedicate the book to scuba divers, with the hope that they will *never* hesitate to call DAN (Diver's Alert Network) at the slightest symptoms of decompression sickness.

Individuals from all walks of life, who have suffered brain injuries, are sometimes our society's forgotten people. This is especially true when they are misdiagnosed and mistreated, and I know how overwhelmed their families can become. Many would benefit from the healing power of hyperbaric oxygen therapy and I dedicate this book to them, in hopes that they can find the treatment they need.

Finally, I dedicate this book to a medical pioneer, and the doctor who gave me back my brain, Dr. Paul G. Harch.

ACKNOWLEDGMENTS

I could fill another volume thanking people who have helped me directly or indirectly on my journey; this book but being one part of it. The list of people that follows is by necessity incomplete. I hope you will understand and forgive me, but when I see you I will thank you in person.

As long as I live, Dr. Paul G. Harch will always be a hero to me, especially because of his dedication to helping suffering patients. His healing hands were the lifeline that dropped into the depths of my mental torment while in the isolation of the county jailhouse, where I sat at the edge of suicide awaiting commitment to the state mental hospital. His is one of the most important voices among those offering profound and substantiated treatment for brain injury through the use of hyperbaric oxygen. His work with not only special needs children and many others, but now also with veterans who suffer from post traumatic stress disorder and traumatic brain injury, deserves nothing less than a Nobel Prize for medicine. I only hope I live long enough to see this occur. To heal a damaged human brain is to restore a life. What more profound healing can there possibly be? I wish him the best with his book, *The Oxygen Revolution.*

My father, mother, and brother stood beside me throughout the darkest hours. They taught me the meaning of unconditional love. Dad, I stayed in the boat like you told me to, and you were right: if we could put a man on the moon, there was surely some help for your son who suffered from brain injury. Mom, your love and compassion is unmatchable, and thanks for asking Dr. Harch to take my case. Ross, there is no greater brother a man could have. Thanks for standing by my side during the toughest times especially when so many others gave up on me, and you helped me get to New Orleans for treatments with Dr. Harch.

My life would be empty without so many true friends, colleagues, fellow recovery people I have known as we trudge the Road of Happy Destiny, fellow Christians, prayer partners, fellow presenters with whom we have had the honor of doing presentations in Edinburgh, Warsaw, the Southwest Disabilities Conference in Albuquerque, New Mexico, Eastern New Mexico University, and in so many other places. As John Donne so aptly stated, "No man is an island...For I am involved in mankind."

Aunt Shirley, I sincerely want to thank you for telling me to go to Dr. Sage. Dr. Sage, thank you for not being in the office that day so I could meet Dr. Jeffrey Beall. Thank you, Dr. Beall, for referring me to Dr. Harch. It was a miracle I ever got to him!

Thank you, Dee Ann, for refusing to give me that beer when I demanded it.

Special thanks go to my spiritual advisors throughout the years: Greg, Harry, and Gary. I also thank all of the wonderful people who have been "trudging the Road of Happy Destiny" with me.

Thanks to the First Baptist Church of Portales, New Mexico, where so many people prayed for me. I want to assure you that your prayers were answered beyond what anyone could have imagined. Because of my successful treatment, the door has been opened for countless others to benefit from the revolutionary healing properties of hyperbaric oxygen therapy.

Thanks to Dr. Michael Shaughnessy of Eastern New Mexico University who taught me everything I know about psychometric assessment procedures, leading me to become a very skilled educational diagnostician for the public schools in New Mexico for fourteen years and now Texas for the past two years. Thanks, too, for pushing me into so many educational research projects, publications, and the additional coursework from George Washington University in the study of brain injury. Thanks also for the early editing you did on the first manuscript.

Lee Ann Hardin, thanks for the prayers, and thanks for never doubting. You were right that God was going to heal me.

Jana and Wanda, you just thought you were hyperbaric technicians. You will always be angels to me.

Virginia McCullough, my book would never have happened without you. I wish you success with *The Oxygen Revolution*. When I grow up, I want to be a writer like you. Thank you for all of your help. God bless you!

Karen Lacey, thank you for the final editing. You are remarkable.

Rusty Oart, you are the real hero, and together we will make sure that this type of tragedy never happens again, especially not to our veterans. You, alongside many other brave veterans, will be the ones to help revolutionize the treatment of brain injury. Not only have you helped to defend the greatest nation on earth, but the advances in the history of neuroscience will be unmatched as each of you, one by one, benefit from HBOT. Like you said, I might have started this, but you are going to put a stop to the misdiagnoses that all too frequently happen.

John Salcedo, God has already started using you to help others by spreading the word about HBOT through your powerful documentaries. I pray for your continued success with *Brain Storm: Oxygen Under Pressure* and *Brain Storm: Signature Wound*. You are a saint for alerting people to the oxygen revolution that will help so many suffering individuals and their families, and thanks for putting Fargo, North Dakota and Frazee, Minnesota, on the map for me.

Finally, despite the fact that we continue to live in a world where terrorists kill innocent civilians, children are born with severe physical and mental impairments, roadside bombs destroy the lives of heroic soldiers and civilians, and greedy, selfish people hold back the progress of mankind all for the sake of making more profit, I still believe in a loving God—one who sent his only Son, Jesus Christ, to not only heal the hopelessly ill in this world but to offer a life everlasting in the next world. I thank God every day for what He has done to help me heal.

Dan L. Greathouse
October 2013

TABLE OF CONTENTS

FOREWORD

Twenty-two years this month. That's how long it has taken to bring this story to publication. A lot has happened in those 22 years, but most importantly the passage of time has allowed reflection on this story and an appreciation for the impact it had on two lives, Dan Greathouses' and mine. Neither Dan nor I in May of 1991 had any idea that a chance meeting facilitated by my old friend and roommate would dramatically and immutably change both of our lives and possibly the lives of untold numbers of people. But, it did. Before you indulge in Dan's astounding life-changing saga you need to know a little bit about the other half of this story which makes Dan's story and our path-crossing even more unbelievable. It is my story, a short story that I have wanted to tell for 22 years.

From the time I was very young I had a yearning to do something significant with my life. I had no idea what it would be, I just hoped it would be something impactful. For a variety of reasons I chose medicine for a career and proceeded to Johns Hopkins University School of Medicine in 1976. Upon graduation I was accepted into the general surgery training program at the University of Colorado, Denver. Three weeks into my internship I was hit by a car in broad daylight and dragged under the car for 50 feet. Witnesses left the scene to avoid seeing "the body" pulled from under the car. When the driver's car jack wouldn't work 16 men from a nearby tennis center lifted the woman's car to pull me unconscious into a waiting paramedic van. Months of hospitalization and multiple surgeries later I hobbled back to my internship and completed two years of training. My surgery days, however, and my dreams of a career in general and plastic surgery, I felt, were over. Needing additional corrective surgery and faced with the likely probability of inability to complete my surgical training I took a medical leave.

After a year of soul-searching I accepted a job offer in New Orleans to work in hospital-based emergency medicine and found my way into a group of physicians who practiced emergency medicine, diving, and undersea medicine. Our center was the central Gulf of Mexico and South Central United States referral center for diving accidents. While interesting, something was missing in my professional life. I had graduated from an excellent medical school with great aspirations. Nine years later I was the class agent who was writing the solicitation letters yearly to my classmates asking for donations to the Annual Fund. All of my classmates had finished their training and were comfortably ensconced in academic careers or medical practices, well on their way to productive fulfilling lives. I, on the other hand, was the Co-Director of the Emergency Department and Hyperbaric Medicine Department in a 150 bed community hospital on the edge of one of the largest swamps in the United States 38 miles from New Orleans. I felt like a complete and total failure in comparison to my classmates. I had not completed a residency, was not yet board certified in any specialty, and was searching for a place in the vast field of medicine. One of my best friends from medical school who was now chairman of the orthopedic department at a large prestigious medical school in New York City came to New Orleans in 1989 for an orthopedic surgeons' convention. I invited him to lunch whereupon he sat down and told me that it was embarrassing to see me engaged in hyperbaric medicine. "Why can't you find a 'respectable' specialty?"

I was angry at the betrayal, rejection, and loss of confidence. It was a devastating repudiation from a "friend" at a time of great internal struggle. Despite the overriding ignorance of the comment, however, it precipitated another round of soul-searching and self-doubt about my future in medicine. Shortly thereafter, I informed the head of our group that I was going to give medicine one more year and if something significant did not happen during that year I was leaving medicine to pursue another line of work. I still had aspirations of making an impact in life, but the reality was that it wasn't happening in medicine.

In the depths of despair I was reminded that I enjoyed hyperbaric medicine and its unappreciated science. I was keenly interested and perplexed by the divers I was seeing with brain decompression sickness, the "bends" of the brain. Poorly appreciated and poorly understood no expert in hyperbaric medicine could answer very simple basic questions about what was going on in the brains of these divers. I decided that my dissatisfaction with my life and career, my predicament, was of my own doing. There was only one solution and that was to change my attitude and follow my interest. I started reading, researching, and asking questions. I delved deeply into all of the old U.S. Navy research on diving and the animal experiments on decompression sickness and air embolism. I was overwhelmed with questions, but no one could answer how divers incurred brain injury, how long or if bubbles were retained in the brain, why the divers in our practice and others weren't cured by the first hyperbaric treatment as the U.S. Navy proclaimed, exactly what were we treating in their brains, how long did we have to treat them, how many treatments did it take to eliminate possible bubbles, and what was the absolute time limit after the accident beyond which treatment would be ineffective.

In the midst of this confusion and void of answers a phone call came from Dr. Jeff Beall. Jeff was my friend, roommate, skiing buddy, and partner for five years in Denver from 1980 to 1985 who was now practicing ENT surgery in northwest New Mexico. Dr. Beall had a diver in his office with major problems, Dan Greathouse. While Dan had been sent to Dr. Beall for "dizziness" from a possible ear injury during diving he recognized that Dan's problems were far more extensive and significant. He called me immediately because he knew I was practicing in the field of diving medicine. I told Jeff that Dan had an air embolism and decompression sickness and needed to be treated immediately. Five days had already passed and the damage was considerable. We succeeded in getting Dan treated with three short hyperbaric oxygen treatments THREE WEEKS LATER; there was no appreciable benefit. Despite my pleas to attempt a lower pressure protocol of hyperbaric therapy that I had just used successfully on a demented diver seven months after his injury the hyperbaric physicians in New Mexico refused.

Months later after the unbelievable saga you will read about in this book, after abandonment by everyone except his parents, after a multiplication of errors and misdiagnoses, I received a phone call from Dan's mother. Dan, in a psychiatric hospital, deeply depressed and despairing of the inability of his physicians to accept his diagnosis of air embolism, was soon to be discharged. I would learn months later that he was planning his suicide upon discharge from the psychiatric facility. I told Betty that he was still treatable and secured his release to my care from the district attorney.

In preparation for Dan's evaluation in New Orleans I had him discontinue all of his antidepressants and psychoactive drugs so that they wouldn't interfere with the electrophysiologic and functional brain imaging tests I had planned. Upon my initial evaluation it was clear and obvious that Dan had a brain injury from diving with his multiple cognitive and neurological findings. Little did I know, however, that this withdrawal of medication would precipitate a depressive crash and state of severe psychomotor retardation (near catatonia) that forced me to admit him to a psychiatric hospital in New Orleans. I remember holding my head in my hands that evening in my office wondering how I could be so crazy as to think that I could bring this young man from a psychiatric hospital and cure him of his malady. I then realized that at the end of the day nothing had changed. His diagnosis was still air embolism and he still had the chance to improve like the demented diver. I persevered and by ambulance ferried him around the city to obtain the tests and see other specialists. At the conclusion of his testing and after a false negative brain blood flow scan on a low resolution scanner I asked his permission for one more test. He assented and I found the highest resolution brain blood flow scanner in New Orleans. It happened to be at a nearby hospital. Upon completion of the scan the radiologist called me and told me that I needed to come and look at Dan's brain scan. He told me he hadn't seen anything like this in a 33-year old man. I did, and in living color at last we could see Dan's diving accident.

I then asked Dan for one last favor, to put him in the hyperbaric chamber at the pressure/dose of oxygen I had used on the demented diver, and then to repeat the brain scan. He agreed. I drove Dan to the hospital for his scan after he exited the hyperbaric chamber. The radiologist read the scan and asked me, "What did you do to him?" I told him and he intoned that this was a remarkable change in his brain. I agreed, and Dan was even feeling a tad better.

I returned to my office and looking out my window reflecting on the previous two week rollercoaster I experienced a most unusual event that I told no one about for many years. It is bizarre, but remains an inexplicable phenomenon, a powerful moving experience that I have withheld telling publicly because of the likely derisive criticisms that would ensue from the medical profession. Now is the time, however. The experience was that I had a very strange open eyes vision as I looked out my office window into the sunset. I could see the next five months of the future as if I was looking down on a play. I was not only in the play, I was the director with total control over the play like the puppetmaster in a marionette. I could see all my actions in the next five months with respect to the treatment and recovery of Dan Greathouse. I saw him progressively and miraculously improving, and recovering function. I had the power to intervene at any time and change the course of events, but I could see that if I just let them unfold with the decisions that I was going to make in the future that it would have the certain outcome in the vision. What was so strange was that this was all in slow motion, yet those future five months passed in 30 seconds or so. It was a bizarre and surreal distortion of time like I had never experienced. It is like the stories that are told in combat or trauma situations where the mayhem, violence, and destruction happens in an instant, but people report a slowing of time, a presence and focus that blocks out the chaos. At the end of it I saw Dan returning to an uproar with sensational claims of a homicidal/suicidal maniac returning to the junior high school. I saw an article in the local newspaper announcing his return to the junior high school. In fact this is exactly what happened and what was recorded in his hometown newspaper. I could lastly see that Dan would surmount this one final hurdle to getting his life back.

The next five months were a time of unparalleled anxious excitement. I KNEW the future for Dan Greathouse because I had SEEN the future. At each step of the way as Dan improved and fulfilled this vision I was bursting with an unconscious anticipation, knowing and having seen the next move and the eventual outcome. Yet, it never occurred to me to tell anyone. I almost doubted the vision. The outcome, however, was certain, as you will read.

Over a year later in another late night conversation with my mother I told her that I had experienced the greatest gratification in my professional life from the experience of helping Dan Greathouse get his life back. I told her that if I died tomorrow I would have felt that my entire life and short career had been a complete success. I could die with no regrets. There was nothing that could surpass this. In repairing Dan's brain injury, a previously untreatable hopeless injury, he was able to recover his cognition, neurological function, musical talent, emotions, relationships, job, life, and future. My mother again reminded me of the fact that I should have died in that car accident many years ago. She was a deeply spiritual and religious person who from the time of my accident felt that there was another plan for me, a plan from a Higher Power. I finally agreed. I now realized what my destiny in life would be.

It is apparent from what you will read in this book that both Dan and I are vehicles, vehicles for the dissemination of the power of this life and quality of life-saving therapy known as hyperbaric oxygen therapy. Our lives seemingly came together by chance, each of us blessed with different talents, but with similar directed missions and purposes in life, both totally outside our choosing and control. What you need to take away from this book is the message that the manner in which this therapy has changed our lives is not unique. Hyperbaric oxygen therapy has the power to transform and give people back their lives like no other therapy known to man. The potential for humankind is nearly limitless, especially when delivered at the time of injury or insult. It is God given and I am honored to be a part of this magnificent plan. Enjoy Dan's amazing story.

Paul G. Harch, M.D.
8/14/2013

PREFACE

Have you ever lost something? Was it important to you? Maybe it was quite valuable, or perhaps even irreplaceable. At one time or another, we've all lost small material things like keys or gloves, and most of us have experienced serious losses, too, from a much-loved pet to a parent to a prized job or business. News reports about earthquakes, wildfires, hurricanes, and tsunamis remind us of catastrophic loss.

I lost something once. It was important to me, intensely personal, and completely my own. I thought, and medical professionals confirmed, that my loss was irreplaceable—it couldn't be recovered. It appeared that acceptance was my only option. As it turned out, though, with the exception of one person, every medical professional I saw misdiagnosed me.

As you probably know, misdiagnoses are common in medicine, and mine is not the first to have had unfortunate results. However, with the knowledge we have today, we can legitimately say that many medical misdiagnoses are avoidable. That belief motivates me to recount the bizarre events that followed the loss of my mental functioning, which was a consequence of "an air embolism and decompression sickness."

Although my particular loss might seem quite unique, it's actually not. Going back to the 1800s, bridge builders were some of the first people to suffer from decompression sickness. At the time, it was known as "caisson disease," because watertight chambers with compressed air were used in the U.S. and Europe in the process of building bridges. Those who suffered from caisson disease experienced paralysis, incoherent speech, dull minds, balance problems, and even death. We now know the symptoms of caisson disease as decompression sickness, and it continued to do its damage until the development of hyperbaric oxygen treatment (HBOT), a treatment that one could legitimately say is the reason I could even write this book.

According to conventional wisdom about using hyperbaric oxygen for decompression sickness, the treatment is most successful when applied immediately upon appearance of the first symptoms, usually within the first twenty-four hours. Until recently, it was believed that after two weeks had passed, the condition was rendered untreatable. (Some physicians who treat divers still believe that.) Well-trained divers are aware of the more subtle symptoms of decompression sickness, including lightheadedness, dizziness, and weakness. What remains true is that we must consider all cases of the sickness as serious, and divers with any of these symptoms must seek immediate medical help.

As you will learn from my story, I'm one of the first people to have been successfully treated for brain decompression illness after a significant delay. I like to say that although I'm not a Nobel Prize winner, and I haven't developed a mathematical or scientific theory that could revolutionize life as we know it, it's quite possible that my case could be famous one day. The story of my successful treatment and recovery has far- reaching implications for all manner of brain injuries, including traumatic brain injuries (TBI) stemming from all causes, such as the common head injuries so many soldiers have suffered in our current wars in Iraq and Afghanistan. Some of these wounds are visible and their resulting disabilities obvious; in other cases, the head injuries are invisible, but just as real. These wounds manifest in maladjustment to society, addictions, inability to cope with family life, post traumatic stress disorder (PTSD), and more.

In fact, as you read my story, I hope you will keep these young men and women in mind, because TBI has enormous implications for individuals and families, and for our society as a whole. Too many returning men and women find themselves unable to adjust and with little hope of a normal life.

In my particular case, the brain injury I sustained would likely have meant that I'd end up living out my days in a mental institution. As you will read, my undiagnosed decompression illness led to stints in psychiatric wards and even days incarcerated in jail like a criminal. For a brief time, I was even suspected of committing a heinous crime. Sadly, life spirals down for many individuals with brain injuries, regardless of the cause. Like Dr. Paul Harch, the medical pioneer who treated me, I believe HBOT can be helpful to many who suffer varying degrees of TBI.

Of the many symptoms from which I suffered with this illness, my mental abilities became significantly dulled, characterized by short-term memory loss and the inability to focus on detail. Because this story contains a great deal of detail, I couldn't have written it (over a period of several years) without help to piece together the sequence of events. I reviewed my father's journal and my mother's notes, along with extensive medical notes that included input from Dr. Paul Harch. I also filled in important information through interviews with my brother and other relatives and friends.

Like everyone else, my life has had any number of dramatic and important events, and some of them make their way into various sections of this book. Three are especially important to my story. One is my continuing recovery from alcoholism through a twelve-step program. My journey to what is now almost twenty-five years of sobriety is a story in itself, and while I refer to it from time to time in this book, it is not the main focus of what I recount here. Without question, my experience with decompression illness, loss of mental abilities, and the dramatic (and frankly, sometimes tragic) aftermath is what, in the end, has motivated me to write this book. I want others to benefit from my experience—it's that simple.

Finally, though, my life as a Christian is what unites all the events of my life, and though my spiritual journey hasn't always been smooth, to say the least, I come back to my Christian beliefs as the anchor for my life.

In terms of vocation—and avocation—my life has long been focused on education. For several years, I taught mathematics and English in the public schools, but I left the teaching trenches to become an educational diagnostician. And, while I'm not a great musician, I continue to write music and perform in a local praise band.

The scuba diving accident in May of 1991 forever changed my life, and this book tells that story. Of course, it's my greatest desire that something in this book offers hope to others who are faced with seemingly impossible barriers and limitations of any kind. So, it is with a great deal of humility that I even begin to offer my story. Countless TBI victims may have even more dramatic stories of hope to share with the world. More than anything, I hope that brain-injured individuals can find the correct diagnosis and treatment before they go through some of what happened to me as a result of ignorance and misconceptions about decompression sickness.

1
TAKING THE PLUNGE

I pursued diving because I'd enjoyed the profound experience of snorkeling for the first time while on a trip to Mexico. One reason I use the word "profound" is because as a child, I was afraid of water, and hadn't overcome that fear and learned to swim until age twelve. The pleasure of snorkeling in Mexican waters served as the trigger that later motivated my interest in pursuing scuba diving.

I had a full life during the years between early sobriety and my diving accident. My recovery from alcoholism, while not always easy, allowed me to pursue a new, stable life. Alcoholism had cost me my marriage and my friends, along with my self-respect and many other valuable things. However, recovery offered me life with the hustle and bustle of teaching during the day at junior high school, working at the night school, playing music on the weekends, and starting graduate classes to work on my administrative degree for the public schools. In fact, my job description at the night school had changed to that of an administrator. I was in the prime of my life, and nothing was going to stop me, or so I believed.

When my thoughts drift back, that time of my life often seems more like a dream than an actual memory. I do recall the day I saw the notice announcing diving classes taught by Sharon Smith, a girls' PE teacher at the same school I taught in. The flyer included a caricature of a funny-looking little man wearing fins and a diving mask and poking his head between the seaweed strands looking at the fish. I thought back to my exciting snorkeling experience in the Yucatan just six months earlier, and I remembered the scuba diving stories a friend had shared. She had painted a beautiful word picture of scuba diving in the Sea of Cortez. Near some of the islands, wild seals would come up next to the divers, almost within arm's length, as they shared their lovely warm Mexican seawater space with the human intruders.

The prospect of a new adventure intrigued me. I had grown up watching countless episodes of underwater adventures with Jacques Cousteau. Somehow, this chance to dive became the ticket to expanding my new life, especially since drinking in dreary smoke-filled barrooms was a thing of the past. For me, life was indeed a playground, and in that spirit I decided to join the scuba diving class.

Sharon, a short, slim, athletic woman, had a determined, drill sergeant demeanor and looked much younger than her actual age. She held the book learning part of the diving lessons in her home, and by showing neat black and white transparencies on an overhead projector, we reviewed information from the lesson book and eventually took written tests. We also had practice dives in a pool.

Diving seemed easy, but now I realize that the materials did not adequately address decompression sickness, commonly called "the bends." The manual included a picture of a hyperbaric chamber used for treatment, along with a paragraph on the illness. Furthermore, we were led to believe that decompression sickness was physically painful, sometimes resulting in unconsciousness. Later, I found out for myself that these facts were only partially true.

I looked forward to open water certification on a spring break trip to San Carlos, Mexico. Unlike the nearby dirty, densely populated city of Guymas, the whitewashed and red tile villas of San Carlos sat next to the blue waters of the Sea of Cortez. Sunlight shimmered on the ocean as waves danced in the distance. The rugged sun-baked lava mountains seemed out of place next to the sea that stretched to the horizon. Several coves and reefs dominated the coastline, and the Sonora Beach, where, incidentally, the movie *Catch 22* had been filmed, was marked by huge powdery sand dunes. The airstrip and several deteriorating buildings were all that remained of the set, which had been constructed to imitate Italy during World War II.

After a stop at the local dive shop, we obtained maps of the nearest dive locations, and we found a place to refill our scuba tanks. Best of all, we also made arrangements for the boat trip to the island of the seals. The divers and sunbathers of our party finally reached Lalo Cove, which nestled between two rocky crags and a stretch of white beach. The cove's smooth waters contrasted with the choppy waves of the distant sea.

"It's time to gear up for the dive," Sharon said to the dive party.

"You bet!" I enthusiastically replied.

Two other experienced divers methodically geared up, making sure to check out their apparatuses as they went along. But I did not use the caution I had been taught. Impulsively, I quickly suited up and was in the water, awaiting the dive instructor. As an aside, I thought I'd landed in paradise! In the company of seven attractive women and only two men, I must have played my cards right.

Time flew once the dive started, and I performed the various underwater tasks for my open water certification. We seemed to rush through the requirements, with no time left for questions. Every task I performed, although I knew I had not done it completely and correctly, was merely checked off the list as "passing."

We continued diving in the cove for the next few days, until I was certified. I enjoyed being in the water so much that I snorkeled between dives. How excited I was as we boarded the chartered boat at the marina on the morning we left for Isla San Pedro, an island known to have many seals and quite possibly the island I'd heard about from my friend.

When we arrived, I noted several seals lounging on the rocks that bordered the water of the small cove. The water was so clear that from the boat we peered well over sixty feet to the bottom. Geared up, I jumped in and swam to the bow of the boat where others in our group had descended a few feet into the Sea of Cortez. Feeling a tug on my fin, I looked down and saw Sharon motioning me to join them in the descent along the anchor line that stretched to the bottom. No sooner had we descended ten or twenty feet when overhead shadows startled me, causing me to almost panic. But then I spotted several seals diving toward us. I had never seen one up close like this, nor had I ever had such an exhilarating experience.

Before my first ascent, I found an old purple, crusted-over conch shell that I recovered with my fin and gently carried by hand to the surface. I remembered my mother's beautiful conch shell from my childhood, although hers was much prettier and very polished. Yet, to this day, I treasure that crusted-over conch shell that I discovered that day at Isla San Pedro.

How was I to know that these days in Mexico would be the last of my diving adventure? Never again would I be allowed this privilege or freedom. I guess it's human nature to wonder if I would have appreciated it even more had I known what would happen later.

At the end of my certification procedures, Sharon presented me with a T-shirt indicating that I had my open water certification. Sometime later, Sharon approached me at school and asked me if I would be interested in a weekend diving trip to Lake Powell. Since the planned trip would be well past my deadlines for graduate work, I quickly agreed to join in the diving party and looked forward to it with great anticipation.

This trip, my second major diving excursion, had ominous signs from the time we got there, including wind picking up on the lake. Then, when I made the first dive, I panicked and swallowed water. Two other men pushed me back to shore. My spirits sank. The cold water of Lake Powell was quite different from the heated pool in the city and the warmer waters of San Carlos. Even with the diving hood, I could not seem to warm up. Something was not right, yet I continued to force my will in the situation. I had the attitude that I was going to dive no matter what!

By the afternoon dive of the first day, I was mentally better prepared for the cold water, but I put my fins on incorrectly and pulled one of the straps completely loose. It fell into murky water, and I panicked and blindly felt around for the lost strap. When I couldn't find it, I took off my gear and hopped into my truck and drove to nearby stores in search of a strap. Looking back on all of this so many years later, I wish to God I had never bothered with that strap. I wish I'd just gone up to camp, borrowed someone's lawn chair and kicked back under a tree somewhere—maybe taken a nap for the rest of the day. I've played out many different scenarios over the years. But just as Captain Ahab pursued Moby Dick with such a monomaniacal passion, I had become this madman with only one thing on my mind. By God, I was going to dive at Lake Powell!

Returning to the ramp, while the others ended their second dive for the day and loaded up equipment to return to camp, I snorkeled in the muddy, shallow water. I felt around for the missing strap, patiently floating in the murkiness until, at last, I found it. How lucky, I thought.

The weather was good the next day, with sun shining brightly in the clear blue morning sky. I was the first one with my gear donned and into the water. Even though, in terms of conditions and preparations, everything looked pretty good, nothing was being done according to the way Sharon had taught us. For example, during my only dive the previous day, we had not paired up as diving partners, and I had a sinking feeling that things were going to go along in the same haphazard way. As well, at no time did I notice anyone using a high altitude dive table to adjust for possible decompression complications. But I dismissed my uneasy sense that something wasn't quite right.

Sharon, unaware of our diving location, was training new divers at a different part at the lake, so I asked another man, Jim, to be my dive buddy and he agreed. But once the dive began, individuals in the group went their own way and Jim didn't wait for me. Even the activity director eventually dove off in his own direction. As any experienced diver will attest, all these slips in protocol are very ill-advised.

When I hit the water, my regulator bubbled strangely, but the activity director yelled from the boat a short distance away that it was okay and to go on. Still I waited, and after the regulator stabilized, I placed it in my mouth and descended into the water, psychologically better prepared this time for the cold. I continued my dive alone near the brightly lit sandstone bottom beneath the boat, hoping my dive buddy would soon join me, or I would join him as soon as I located him. Finally, the others entered the water, and the activity director swam rapidly by. I tried in vain to catch up as he dove down a ravine to a cliff and disappeared into the depths.

Because of a kind of premonition, I did not follow the others into the deep. I swam back up the ravine toward the flat sandstone bottom below the boat. However, I then convinced myself to return back down the ravine in hopes of finding the others. I was alone in the water and could not see anyone. Once again, I dove down the rocky ravine toward the edge of the abyss, and once again, after seeing none of the dive party, I returned back up the ravine toward the boat.

I swam along the flat sandstone plateau just under the boat, and then Jim went past me in the clear cold water. I tried to catch up with him, and that is when the accident happened. My regulator began to free flow, and a steady stream of compressed air rushed into my mouth and lungs. I panicked, but even though I couldn't think clearly, I knew if I left the regulator in my mouth, my lungs would expand until they exploded like balloons.

I jerked the regulator from my mouth. Completely overcome with panic by this time, what little scuba training I had, along with any ability to reason, left me. I stupidly grabbed for the secondary regulator and placed it to my mouth. Of course, I could draw no air through it because all of the air was rushing through the first regulator.

Sharon had trained me in all of these matters, first at the pool in the city, and then in my open water dive certification in San Carlos, Mexico. But I panicked anyway, although many correct ways out of this situation exist. Because of my distress, I quickly ran out of time. Had I been following safety precautions in the first place, I would not have gone on this dive without my buddy nearby, a dive plan, and high altitude dive chart adjustments.

Looking back on my predicament with the free flow regulator, I could have hooked the regulator in the side of my mouth and continued with a slow ascent. Probably my best bet would have been ascending while exhaling the newly taken in compressed air from my body, as I made a controlled ascent to the surface. Had I been with an experienced dive buddy, I could have made a safe ascent with him, taking turns using his regulator. So much for the diving buddy option, as my diving partner was nowhere around.

I did neither of the two safe ascent options at my disposal, and instead, did the worst possible thing. The accident happened subtly and quietly, without drama or obvious signs. Car crashes and gun shootings have noisy immediacy. My accident began when I started the ascent. I let out one small bubble of air, and I remember that bubble racing ahead of me toward the surface. I could see the sky up through the water. I pushed my fins off the sandstone, thrusting myself upward. I held my breath as tightly as possible, not letting *any* air escape from my lungs. As I ascended, I braced myself for a blackout which I had been taught could happen with the bends.

After surfacing in the bright sunlight, I let the air out from my lungs in a huge sigh of relief and happily noted that everything seemed to be okay. Dr. Paul Harch, whom you will come to know later in the book, explained that I'd had an air embolism. To be technically correct, I had decompression illness, which includes air embolism and decompression sickness, and occurred when I held my breath and came to the surface. An air embolism happens as bubbles of air occur in the heart or vascular system. My bloodstream had been infused with different types of gasses, including oxygen and nitrogen. I had not used any altitude corrections, and the bubbles that were released by the air embolism then also absorbed gas from all the rest of my body tissues, causing bigger bubbles and bigger problems.

When it came time to leave for the marina, I got back into the boat with the others. As we approached the marina, we were pulled over by a patrol boat and the activity director was cited for not having a current boat license. Luckily avoiding expensive fines, he was only given a warning when he convinced the officer that the license had been sent for but not yet received. We proceeded to hitch up the boat at the dock to get tanks filled for the afternoon dive. I still had not experienced any noticeable symptoms and prepared for the dive at Castle Rock.

Because of some growing fatigue, which I quickly attributed to being overworked from the school year and the busy weekend, I did not dive very long or very deep even though my regulator was functioning normally. I remember stopping to rest on a large rock jutting out of the water and having a slight problem keeping my balance, but I didn't think of it as a symptom.

Later, Dr. Harch conducted many tests and discovered that the bubbles had somehow travelled to my brain because of what he believed to be a physiological anomaly unique to me. What I told Dr. Harch at the time and what I remember now differ in some ways. Initially, I told Dr. Harch that while on the second dive, I felt extremely fatigued. I got out of the water and sat in the rocky beach. I talked with the dive instructors. "God, I'm exhausted. I don't feel right. Is this what they describe as decompression sickness?"

One of the instructors replied, "No, you are fat and out of shape, diving at altitude in cold water. You need to get back in the water."

Eventually, I went back into the water, and I actually felt somewhat better. In fact, the fatigue seemed to go away. Dr. Harch later explained that that was classic for decompression sickness. In other words, recompressing myself under water would probably help me feel better. Since I had not blacked out, nor did I have any pain in my joints, I happily concluded that I'd avoided decompression sickness. Completely unaware that the silent, seemingly uneventful accident had already occurred, I instead had sighed with relief. I was quite grateful to have reached the safety of the surface despite the terrifying ascent. However, I'd actually set into motion the events that would forever change my life.

For the rest of the day I felt grateful that I'd avoided decompression sickness and happily joined the others for a pizza dinner. Conversation was lively in the early evening light, and after we ate, Sharon, who had hopefully been teaching all of the important diving rules to her classes at the other side of the lake that day, signed the beginners' logbooks and presented the awards of certification for the new open water divers. Looking back, it seems that although training appeared to be cursory, festivities were paramount. For me, the true nightmare had just begun.

2
THE LONG JOURNEY BEGINS

Subtle symptoms began on the drive home from Arizona to New Mexico. After piecing together the events, though, I know I had only had the first glimmer of understanding. Even in retrospect, nothing particularly drastic occurred at first. For example, as I drove, I felt as if my body was thrown further around the curve than the actual path of my truck. This distorted my physical perception of my body in space. The *proprioceptive* senses involve the brain's ability to know where the body is in the three dimensional experience, and these senses also involve balance. My decompression illness interfered with my spatial perception.

The only thing I can liken it to was my experience driving drunk many years before—an experience that taught me how alcohol distorted sensory responses. Now, coming back from Arizona, but not under the influence of alcohol, I had difficulty keeping the truck on the road when I navigated the curves. The sensation was subtle, and since the road didn't have that many curving sections, I had little trouble for most of the trip.

One odd incident stands out, however. I ran over a piece of lumber on the highway that under ordinary circumstances I could have easily dodged with a quick adjustment of the steering wheel. If I'd been able to do that, I'd have easily avoided what happened next. When my right rear tire hit the wood, I heard a loud thump, and as I slowed to a halt, I could hear air escaping from the tire—a most inconvenient flat. I recall being irritable and having difficulty working with my tire jack. Luckily, one of the younger boys traveling in the dive caravan stopped to help me. Still, little things upset me, like briefly losing a nut in the sand at the edge of the road.

Much later, after the damage of the diving accident had become all too apparent, Dr. Harch reviewed some less obvious details surrounding the events. For example, after leaving the lake, I drove up seven hundred feet to get out of the park; ascending in altitude is one of the worst things to do after a scuba diving accident. Even worse, to get back home I had to drive over a 7,000 foot mountain pass. It was when I came down the other side of the pass that I was unable to avoid the piece of lumber in the road. Even more revealing to Dr. Harch, I couldn't assemble my tire jack.

Dr. Harch knew immediately that decompression sickness was involved in these "lapses." I recall him saying, "Give me a break. Here's a person who played keyboard and guitar, and all of a sudden he can't assemble a jack?"

It's a well known fact that people who fly right after a diving excursion are at increased risk for developing decompression sickness. That 7,000 foot pass could be likened to taking an airline flight.

As soon as we arrived at Sharon's home, I began to unload air tanks and scuba gear. My legs were somewhat "surprised" several times by the uneven asphalt and more than once I nearly stumbled. Must be fatigue, I thought. Nothing that a good night's sleep wouldn't take care of.

What a shock the next morning when I teetered slightly off balance as I walked the short distance from my bed to the bathroom. But I still didn't feel alarmed enough to suspect anything. Somehow, it stuck in my mind that because I had not become unconscious or developed pain in my joints, nothing serious had occurred. It never even entered my mind to call DAN (the Divers' Alert Network).

I taught that day at the junior high school and then showed up to supervise the night school. It was then that I learned that my house had been broken into and vandalized. Germain, my roommate, called to give me the news, which sidetracked me from the balance problems and continuing fatigue. Germain had come to live with me when he was sobering up and attempting to get his life together. Divorced with three boys, he held down a job, and my house gave him a relatively inexpensive place to call home, at least for a while.

Later, I found his behavior a bit suspicious. Something sounded odd about Germain's description of the event, and it piqued my curiosity. He had only a few things stolen, while I had many valuable items missing. That fact alone certainly sowed some seeds of doubt.

Nonetheless, my physical symptoms continued, and not wanting to overreact, I began to blame my problems on my inner ear, one of the body's mechanisms involved in maintaining balance. My mother first suggested that possibility, and Sharon, my diving instructor, supported her speculation.

What still remains inexplicable was the fact that a diving instructor would not connect the symptoms I reported with decompression sickness and urge me to contact DAN. Looking back now, I wish I had called DAN immediately. This inner ear hypothesis would later turn out to be the red herring in my medical case, but at the time it seemed like an entirely plausible explanation. Besides, since I was afraid of decompression sickness, I reassured myself that everything was going to be all right.

Still, the weaving continued. One of my colleagues even mentioned it, and when I told him what had happened, he linked the symptom with diving. I approached Sharon again, suggesting to her that I might have decompression sickness. She continued to maintain that it was just an inner ear problem.

Only at my mother's insistence, did I agree to see a doctor to have my "inner ear problem" checked out. I saw Dr. Jeffrey Beall, a specialist in matters of the ear, and a man with a soothing bedside manner and calm voice. Dr. Beall also doubted that I had decompression sickness, and he gave me standard tests to assess my inner ear and to check for equal pressure between the inner and outer ear. Although everything appeared normal, he prescribed histamine to increase the blood flow to any possible damaged areas of the inner ear, allowing it to repair itself. He scheduled a follow-up appointment for two weeks later. I found it difficult to drive home from his office.

Meanwhile, I went off on an already planned rafting trip with a couple of good friends, Timothy and Bill. Our families had crossed paths over the years, the way families do in the tapestry of small town life. I had regained some of the threads in this tapestry after I sobered up, and these friends were among those who helped me during that time.

So, I went away for my grand rafting adventure despite some significant warning signs that something was seriously wrong.

We planned our trip to take us down the Animas River back to Farmington. While I continued to feel out of balance, my thought processes were fine. I had to be extremely careful not to fall from the river bank or off the raft itself into the river. We wore helmets and lifejackets in preparation to ride the late spring runoff that Timothy described as rocking-and-a-rolling. The water was swift and extremely cold, a challenge for a three-man rafting crew and I'd been on a raft only one other time.

Starting out, the sun shone brightly, and we weren't yet plagued by the oppressive heat that only the southwest desert can generate. The river twisted and turned, always following the path of least resistance. Sometimes it flowed smoothly and calmly, and other times it gushed quickly over rocks and medium sized rapids. The sun heated the surrounding sandstone cliffs and rocky hills, and the colors of spring life splashed the canvas of reality with the variety of divine genius. No artist's canvas would ever capture the diversity and complexity of the river and its surrounding valley. We often spotted deer and other animals from our little rubber raft.

I remember thinking that life was a lot like the river trip, with so many hazards and unexpected turns. We never really know what's ahead, but we keep on floating down the river, placing our fate in the flowing current. Before long, our three-man crew had to heed some warning signs about a dangerous diversion dam. The signs didn't kindly suggest getting out of the river; they demanded that we travelers disembark immediately.

We paddled to the shore so we could carry the raft around the dam. As soon as I stood and began to help move the raft, I was reminded of my balance problem. How annoying! As usual, I wondered just how soon this situation would correct itself, but I faithfully took the histamine Dr. Beall had prescribed. I had a good time that day, but not too long after, I thought about the river and wondered if my memories of the trip would be my last thoughts before my death. I didn't know it at the time, but everything in my life would soon unravel.

On the trip I had flashes that things were not as they should be, including bouts of forgetfulness. That was easily dismissed as exhaustion from the long river rafting adventure, but these seemingly small events were the start of more serious memory issues. Dr. Harch has since told me that exhaustion and memory problems are common symptoms in decompression sickness and other forms of brain injury.

Later that week, my mother was shocked to hear my slurring speech. She had my brother call me to see if he could detect it, too. Had she not known me better, she would have sworn I was drunk. Everything had gotten worse—my balance, memory, fatigue, and irritability. I jokingly, but really somewhat seriously, quipped to a colleague at work that I'd use a gun on myself because I couldn't go on like this.

A few days later, I ranted and raved in the teachers' lounge at school, offending a colleague who had been a former roommate. But in the moment, I didn't care. This kind of emotional outburst and general short temperedness is common with brain decompression sickness—and other forms of TBI and PTSD. Losing the ability to concentrate, which started around that time, is common as well. Before long, I started resting on the floor in front of my class during the last period of the day. I had *never* been this tired before.

One morning, I was in the middle of completing some award certificates for a handful of exemplary math students, when I couldn't form the letters of the words. My brain knew exactly what letter to form, but my fingers couldn't complete the eye-to-hand fine motor integration. As my hand moved to form a specific letter, something entirely different appeared on the paper. This happened again and again, making me increasingly alarmed. I completed the certificates, but I had to concentrate hard on each minute hand movement required to write the letters.

When I talked to Sharon about it later, she said, "Those inner ear things can sure be tricky."

By this time, I found her dismissive responses to me empty and useless. I never approached her again about any of my symptoms. What I needed was medical help. Deep in my heart I knew this was not some sort of inner ear problem.

While waiting during the two weeks for the follow-up appointment with Dr. Beall, the symptoms mounted and became more shocking. Just how far would this progress? Because of my deteriorating situation, I went to see my family physician, Dr. Rhine, who had helped during my early recovery from alcoholism. I didn't know Dr. Beall well, and besides, he was an ear, nose, and throat doctor. I was absolutely convinced that Dr. Rhine could help me get to the bottom of my dilemma. During my appointment with Dr. Rhine, I attempted to explain the incident at Lake Powell and my current symptoms, but the story had become increasingly difficult to tell.

"I rather doubt that you have the bends," he said, using the common divers' term.

Despite his words, I went over the symptoms again, finding myself fighting for the words to express myself. Somehow, though, it all boiled down to a single symptom, dizziness. He prescribed a medication to treat dizzy spells, but then he alarmed me by saying that he wanted an MRI (magnetic resonance imaging) of my brain if things did not improve in two weeks.

I distinctly remember him raising his eyebrows when I told him about my difficulty filling out the award certificates at school. He also confirmed my deepest growing fear that difficulties with writing were not usually associated with inner ear problems. *So, something* is *really wrong with me*, I thought. *I knew it!*

The waiting had begun to get to me. First, Dr. Beall wanted me to wait two weeks before returning to him. Now, Dr. Rhine wanted me to wait two weeks before coming back to him for an MRI. I wanted some answers. My fear of the unknown grew stronger, and the terrifying possibility of a brain tumor loomed in my mind. I felt as if a black widow spider had eaten a hole in my brain and made itself a comfortable new home within the deteriorating matter contained in my skull.

When I came back from seeing Dr. Rhine, I decided that I needed a more spiritual approach to my problem, since the medical world was doing little to comfort me. Meanwhile, I encountered more problems with Germain. He'd illegally hooked up the cable outside of my home to get free TV, and I went outside and disconnected it. That upset him and he demanded an explanation.

I explained that honesty was a big part of my alcoholism recovery program, and enjoying cable TV without paying for it didn't fit a life based on honesty. Germain told me that honesty was no longer important to him, and he'd already re-hooked the cable.

My temper was no longer within my control, and I wasn't going to let some drunken jerk live in my house and tell me how things were going to be. I ordered him out of my house, and I had some extra money for him to use as a deposit for another apartment. Germain laughed, and then made fun of my slurred speech and balance problem. I don't know what kept me from hitting him square in the jaw, but fortunately, I was able to restrain myself. Ironically, a year or so later, I learned that Germain was experiencing his own medical problems—much worse than mine.

The next weekend, Peggy, a good friend from graduate school, and I drove out to Canyon DeChelly for a three-day spiritual gathering of recovery groups of various kinds. I took along my guitar for sing-alongs by the campfires at night. Peggy did most of the driving to the beautiful ancient

Anasazi ruins. We made camp at the mouth of the canyon amidst the towering cottonwood trees. We were all survivors of the serious grip of alcohol, and had come together to celebrate life. Difficult symptoms aside, I intended to enjoy the fellowship of a positive group of people.

The next morning, tapping on the window of my truck awakened me. I smiled at the sight of an old friend I hadn't seen in years. The last time I had seen Ron, I took him to a Native American alcohol treatment center on the western side of the state. Sadly, he'd continued in a downward cycle, but there he was at my camper shell window early one Arizona morning.

I was overjoyed to see him, and he reported with excitement that he'd been sober for more than a year and he'd hoped to see me at this gathering. I explained that health issues caused my problems with speech and balance—and I hadn't started drinking again! The weekend was a positive time for all of us and my spirits lifted.

One of the days, we hiked down to the bottom of Canyon DeChelly. Ron and Peggy had to help me down into the canyon because of the balance problems, but along the way I found an old shepherd's staff and that gave me more stability. I took the staff home as a reminder of that enchanting day of gratitude, sobriety, and spirituality. Despite my problems, I felt very close to God and grateful to be with Ron, my one-year-sober friend. Yes, it seemed that God did perform miracles.

Sadly, when we sat around the campfire after our hike, my guitar felt much different in my hands and I couldn't play as well as I had before. My voice sounded different, even weak. I put away the guitar and listened to the others play and sing. I wouldn't pick up the guitar again for many months.

The next morning I was so exhausted that I asked Peggy if she would mind returning home a day early. Fortunately, she was fine with a new plan.

My deterioration escalated. All ordinary tasks of life that I had previously completed with little effort were now seemingly impossible, demanding chores. Writing, playing the guitar and piano, once important to me, were all performed only with great effort. I became angry that I could no longer play simple, familiar pieces. I would practice over and over and over, and the result would be the same. I no longer had control of my fingers to play the correct notes. My mind knew what to do, but my fingers reacted another way. Soon, I could no longer console myself that this would all turn around, that it was only a matter of time.

About this time, Lawrence, an acquaintance of mine, visited me. He'd done some carpentry work for me the summer before, converting a work shed into an air-conditioned music studio. He needed the money, and I needed the music studio. Lawrence had several more years of sobriety under his belt than I. A welder by trade, he preferred welding art projects to practical welding jobs. He created many interesting Native American style metal sculptures of all sizes. Lawrence's calm nature and outlook were reassuring amidst the chaos I was experiencing. One night, he was with me in the car when I was driving. I knew he was anxious when I almost missed a curve in the road, but he tried to laugh it off and not upset me. I believe, though, that he knew that something was wrong with me.

Slowly, painfully, I was losing friends and generally withdrawing. Sinister feelings of impending doom crowded into my life. We say in New Mexico that the sun shines brightly in the Land of Enchantment. But the golden rays no longer shared my home.

With Germain gone—finally—the house was empty. I desperately needed to complete the school year, and tried to settle down and focus on this goal. In normal times this would have been a minor event, but it had expanded into a Herculean task. I began to doubt I could do it, especially when I still had to rest on the floor during my sixth period class. Fortunately, my students continued to behave, because I had a strict discipline policy. The kids didn't want to cross the line and then have to stay after school to listen to the shrieking sounds of opera music. I also had gained a great deal of respect by sponsoring support groups for many of the troubled students.

I prepared my lessons and showed them on the overhead projector with the help of a student because I simply couldn't do it alone. I was utterly exhausted. Luckily, I had no more graduate classes until either late in the summer or the next fall, and only one music gig was on the horizon.

I desperately needed a breather, but I knew in my heart that I was experiencing more than exhaustion. I continued to believe decompression illness was the root of my problems, but since I'd begun to lose the ability to think clearly, I didn't know what to believe about what everyone insisted was *not* decompression illness. It's difficult to describe how I felt. I can say that while I certainly hadn't started drinking again, I felt like I had the worst hangover of my life. My thoughts had become dull, my reaction time had slowed, and my short-term memory was skittish.

I even forgot to do my morning meditations, although it seemed that I carried on a conversation with God each and every minute because I was afraid. I'd already talked with my diving instructor and two medical doctors, but no one confirmed my suspicions about decompression sickness. If I'd been thinking clearly I'd have skipped all of these people and just called DAN for professional help, what I should have done in the first place. But the fear of actually suffering from decompression sickness had a tight grip on me.

I also sensed something deeply psychological was taking over, but I dismissed these thoughts because of the mental, spiritual, and emotional work I had done in my efforts to maintain my sobriety. I was experienced in dealing with life without alcohol, and I'd also quit smoking and survived a divorce.

Although I had decided against taking the medication Dr. Rhine had prescribed for my dizziness, one morning I felt particularly tired, though I'd slept many hours. I drank several cups of coffee and took the medication. Later, after I arrived at school, my body experienced a rush of heat. Sweat beads formed on my forehead and a drop of blood dripped from my nose.

I stood in one spot and shuddered. Then, a wave of nausea gripped me. Looking back, I know I felt shaken, as if something had happened in my brain. Yet, I wasn't willing to confront this new event. I tried to forget it, rationalizing that I'd had too much coffee. That's what caused the reaction to the medication, I told myself.

A few hours later, I heard a commotion in the hallway and went to see what was going on. Bill Barker, the assistant principal, was physically forcing a young seventh grade girl out of the building. The air resounded with yelling, screaming, and the young girl's sobbing. I couldn't believe my eyes and ears. As Bill, a muscular ex-marine, and the girl passed my open doorway, she called out my name.

"Mr. Greathouse, Mr. Greathouse, please help me," she screamed between sobs and gasps.

I then recognized the girl. Marie was one of my students who attended a support group at the school and had been in some trouble before. It looked as if Bill was kicking her out of school right in broad daylight and in front of us all. My students were upset, but I stood there like a powerless idiot, unable to formulate my thoughts. I couldn't comfort Marie, a petite, nonviolent student. She had some problems, but nothing that warranted Bill's military-type response.

Even today, I can hear Marie's voice calling out to me for help. I wish to God I'd had my wits about me and been able to intervene, but I was frozen, not by fear, but by some debilitating process. Of course, if I had been thinking clearly, I would have called protective services and reported the violent way Bill abused this girl. I can only say that it felt so awful to know that what was going on in front of my eyes was wrong, yet be powerless to do anything to stop it; much like what was going on in my own body.

3
FIGHTING FOR TREATMENT

During this stressful time, I had nightly telephone conversations with my mother, who heard my speech difficulties and confirmed them with my brother. Apparently, she harbored some fear that I may have started drinking again. My parents, Jack and Betty Greathouse, are religious people, but they're also practical and good problem solvers—and they never give up when faced with a challenge.

Initially, they encouraged me to be patient and wait for this problem to correct itself, but eventually doubt set in. Although my mother was a teacher and had an interest in science, she knew nothing about decompression sickness. Finally, Mom made arrangements to fly up to Farmington to check on me after my difficulties with balance and gait hadn't resolved. The prescriptions had all proven worthless. Her trip to see me initiated her journey into my nightmare.

About this time, a student of mine, Paula, came to my room to visit with me. Paula was another one of my students who attended one of the support groups for troubled junior high school students. She'd had a tough background, but I always remember her façade of seventh grade optimism about life. I guess the best way to describe her situation is to say that since her parents fought all the time, the police were as much a part of her life as football was for the more fortunate junior high school kids.

When Paula came to see me, I had a feeling that she had come to talk with me about her friend, Marie. She was concerned, because Marie had been kicked out of school.

I remained calm and listened, but had little to offer other than pat answers. Had I not been so ill, I would have focused on the issue at hand. Because of what happened to Marie, Paula announced that she intended to quit school and she spoke with great agitation—for a long time. That was okay, because I needed time to form an intelligent answer. In the end, I was able to talk her into coming back to school the next fall. Over the previous years, I had developed a reputation for handling discipline in various creative ways, and that day Paula thanked me for listening and wished me a good summer. I had managed to get through one more day with my students and still accomplish something.

Ironically, the way things were going, I was not certain that *I* would be back in the fall. I wavered about many things, but I continued to attempt to live one day at a time.

After observing me for only one day, my mother prompted me to make the phone call that should have been made weeks ago—the call to DAN. She actually made the call herself since I had trouble dialing numbers and talking with people, especially after a long day. Through the hotline, I learned about a Dr. Dellarosa, located in the metropolitan area of the Rio Grande Corridor. But as fate would have it, he was out of the country—on a scuba diving trip!

I spoke with a friendly and helpful nurse named Charlotte. With my mother listening on the other phone, I answered questions about my diving trip. Charlotte was alarmed that I had waited so long to call DAN and even indicated that most likely nothing could be done for me this late. For successful recovery, decompression sickness had to be treated almost immediately. As I've said, that was the standard belief at the time and remains so in many circles. My spirits sank to a new low. Why had I not immediately called that first morning after returning from the trip? What in the world was I thinking? Later, Dr. Harch told me that all of this was a sign of clouded judgment, a common symptom associated with decompression sickness.

My self-blame intensified, and soon I thought I *deserved* everything that was going on now because I had been so stupid and not called DAN sooner. I continued in a state of shock and disbelief that I'd not understood decompression illness and the use of hyperbaric oxygen treatment. I had been afraid to move on to the only logical treatment for my symptoms, hoping that my difficulties were just an inner-ear-related problem. It's strange how one can choose to be in denial.

As the conversation with Charlotte, the DAN nurse, continued, I rationalized my actions in hopes of quelling the rising fear in the pit of my stomach—a fear that grew quickly. I went over and over the details of my dive at Lake Powell. I could not quit replaying it in my mind. Meanwhile, my mother took notes as I listened to Charlotte through the intensifying and crushing mental numbness.

Something was said about going to Albuquerque. Something was said about leaving immediately. Something else was said about an MRI and meeting with a Dr. Barnett, a neurologist. We were to leave tonight so that we could be there early in the morning. Had my mother not been there to carry on the telephone conversation and take notes, I would have missed the important information. As it turned out, I no longer had the motor coordination necessary to drive two hundred miles, so she would have to take me.

My mother's spirits had lifted because at least we were heading in the direction of expert medical advice, and I'd have an MRI to determine the extent of my brain damage. During the drive, I attempted to meditate on what my brain might look like in the pictures that would be obtained from the MRI. I thought back to what I learned in high school and through my own human anatomy studies. My recollection was that the cerebellum was the portion of the brain associated with balance.

Acting like I had it together, I thanked my mom for coming up to check on me and for driving with me to see a neurologist so far away. At one point, I told my mother that I would take over the driving, but that didn't last long. Attempting to stay on the road, I began weaving, unable to steer the car properly. This gave me a hint of the limitations I faced. I became upset, but I was more fatigued than anything. Needless to say, Mom took back over the driving.

That night in my hotel room, I realized how much I preferred sleeping over being awake. During sleep I didn't have to worry about balance or driving or slurring my speech. The only problem was that sooner or later I would have to wake up to the same nagging symptoms, and I never felt truly rested even after a full night's sleep.

The next morning, my mother and I ate breakfast at a diner. I immediately noted that I could barely carry on a conversation or lift a cup of coffee without great difficulty—more loss of fine motor skills and control, as if I had a short in my wiring. I had to consciously think out every step of handling a cup or a fork. Even then, I spilled coffee and choked as I swallowed. Every sentence I spoke required careful thought, too, and that led to speaking less—something my brother noted later. I had always been a talkative sort, and my periods of silence struck my brother as quite uncharacteristic.

I feared the effects of the stressful situation on my mother—despite her ability to maintain her calm composure. She'd always found her strength in our family. I, on the other hand, had drifted from the family. When I'd sobered up, I found I could no longer be around some of my relatives because they drank, and a few drank to excess. Drinking had resulted in verbally and sometimes physically abusive situations. I'd had difficulty adhering to the adage to "live and let live." But some relatives would be meeting us here in Albuquerque, and while I didn't welcome that, my mother needed their support. Looking back, I know that spending time with me was no picnic.

The MRI itself made me fearful, especially after entering the dark and initially silent massive MRI machine. I wondered if the inside of my coffin would be like this, but I was startled when the machine abruptly began a steady jackhammer sound as the imaging of my brain was conducted.

Even though I have no proof of a literal hell, there is definitely a hell on earth. The waiting room at Dr. Barnett's office offered glimpses of the hell of brain injury—babies with brain damage sustained during birth, a young woman with a brain tumor, an older woman afflicted with Alzheimer's disease. I felt like a prisoner and feared that offices like this would define my future.

My visions of a troubled future made Dr. Barnett's words even more shocking. "I can't find anything wrong with your brain."

"Really?" I said. "I can't believe it! You've just made me the happiest man in the world!" That was my first reaction.

Although none of my neurological symptoms had disappeared, I was relieved that I didn't have a brain tumor, multiple sclerosis, or some other nervous system disorder. The doctor continued listing things he had ruled out. Dr. Barnett also said that none of the neurological problems were related to diving. In fact, he attributed my symptoms to a sinus problem that showed up on the MRI. He suggested that I return to Dr. Beall, whose two week follow-up appointment with me just happened to be the next day. I could hardly believe my ears! So, this was not as bad as I had imagined.

I have had many sinus problems in my life, but never had I been this sick before. Even though I was doubtful that my problem was a simple sinus infection, I returned home to visit with Dr. Beall once again, only to be told that no such sinus problem was present. I reported to him that the histamine had provided no improvement in my balance, and he looked at the MRI scans from Albuquerque. He mentioned his good friend, Paul Harch, a doctor in New Orleans who might be able to help me. But, because I didn't feel good about Dr. Beall's approach, I didn't take his advice at that point. After all, hadn't he given me medication that hadn't helped? Actually, I was in no position to make these decisions, because my thinking and mental processes were noticeably dull. I left his office more confused and very discouraged.

Behind the scenes, however, Dr. Harch and Dr. Beall had an important phone conversation. Dr. Harch dismissed the idea that my symptoms were related to the inner ear. Based on his expertise in diving medicine, he told him that I had an air embolism and brain decompression sickness. I needed to have hyperbaric therapy immediately. Dr. Harch wanted a brain-blood-flow scan because he believed that it would reveal evidence of the decompression sickness. He recommended to the doctor for me to get to the nearest hyperbaric chamber in New Mexico. At the time, the state had only one hospital with a chamber. Dr. Harch contacted colleagues there and explained my case; however, my treatments were delayed for another two weeks. This is one of the many times that Dr. Harch became livid over issues related to so many patients' limited access to appropriate HBOT. We later learned the delays were caused by the Albuquerque hyperbaric facility's effort to verify that I had insurance to cover the treatment so long after the accident. Although I didn't realize it at the time, and I learned about this much later, there were some attempts to make arrangements for hyperbaric treatments, even though I was outside the window of opportunity for treatment.

Then the waiting game began for my first HBOT treatments. My mother, who was staying with me because of my deteriorating condition, handled most of the phone calls and took down many notes. Most of it confused me—Dr. this or Dr. that in New Mexico or New Orleans. It all ran together. So many opinions and disagreements about what treatment could help. Over and over, my hopes were dashed on the rocks of endless waiting for some distant phone call from some distant who-the-hell-knows what doctor. Of course, none of my symptoms improved, and in fact, only worsened. I could feel my mental condition deteriorating as each minute passed, and my house became a prison cell.

Old friends called, and one visited. I overheard little scraps of what my mother said to people from my past—the people all mixed together in my mind and seemed like strangers anyway. "I'm not sure what to do . . . could you please come up here so I can leave? I need a break. He's just too much for me to handle" . . . and then she would quietly cry. Although I'd forget her words and not understand what she meant, I never forgot the sound of her crying.

Finally, after obtaining approval from the insurance company, there would be further neurological tests followed by three hyperbaric treatments, and then there would be the same neurological tests to determine if there had been any improvement. We were cautioned that if there was no improvement in my condition, the treatments would be discontinued. The insurance company required specific guidelines for treatment and then they'd make a decision about their effectiveness. At the back of this book, you'll find a website for DAN, where you can read current guidelines for hyperbaric treatment following a diving accident. Ultimately, however, the decision about *delayed* hyperbaric treatment following a diving accident is up to the doctor involved. Some doctors will no doubt maintain that it isn't worth trying after a 24-hour period, or they may not have heard of the great advances in hyperbaric medicine. For these reasons, I believe divers should question their family physicians about their beliefs concerning HBOT as an appropriate treatment for all kinds of brain injuries.

Dr. Harch believed in delayed treatment based on his experience with a diver he had successfully treated a full five months after the diving accident. The diver was recompressed and then treated at a lower pressure. Dr. Harch, continuing to work behind the scenes all this time, had called and pleaded with the New Mexico doctors to get me into a chamber as soon as possible. He wanted them to treat me as he had done with the other diver. Sadly, these doctors told Dr. Harch that his suggestion was crazy and that there was no established and accepted precedent for it. Well, of course, Dr. Harch knew that, but he had tried the treatment and it worked.

I learned that the New Mexico doctors had called Duke University and DAN and discussed Dr. Harch's treatment idea. These "experts" also said that it was "just crazy." But despite this disbelief, the New Mexico docs agreed with the stipulation that I should have only three hyperbaric treatments and if I didn't improve, that would be the end of it.

Once again, my mother and I went back to Albuquerque. We made arrangements to stay with relatives in their beautiful home in the foothills of the Sandia Mountains. While the surroundings were quite beautiful, it was here that I would learn once again the truth to Shakespeare's adage: "A little more than kin and a little less than kind." Most of this ugliness revolved around resentment among some relatives that my decision to stop drinking had driven a wedge between us—not an uncommon occurrence when one person in a family or group changes.

It was incredibly ironic that I had worked so hard to stay sober, only to find myself feeling either drunk or hungover all the time. I walked like a drunk, and my speech was slurred as though I had been drinking. In addition to this, my emotional swings reminded me of emotional swings I had experienced during my later drinking days.

I grew angry and irritable through all this and then had relatives lecturing me about my supposed outbursts. Dr. Harch has since told me that these outbursts are classic symptoms of brain injury. Still, the suggestion that my problems were purely psychological was silly and fed my anger. Besides, I wanted to leave, but wasn't able to drive across town, much less two hundred miles.

At one point, I came close to picking up that first drink, but I believe the hand of God intervened. I was spared the ordeal of a slip and ruining over two years of recovery. On a purely practical level, if I had begun to drink again, I would have introduced a complicating variable into the equation of my undiagnosed condition. And, it would have overshadowed all other aspects of my symptoms, because I would have entered a phase of continued drunkenness, from which I might not ever have escaped. It would then have been so easy for all the doctors and family members to just write me off with the simple diagnosis of "town drunk." I doubt I would have lived very long.

I often wonder, and Dr. Harch also asks, just how many homeless people (and prison inmates) who suffer from drug and alcohol addiction, mental illnesses, and other anti-social behavior are actually the victims of some undiagnosed mild (at the very least) traumatic brain injury.

During that time, I had the initial one full day of neurological testing, which happened to be at Dr. Barnett's office. From Beall to Barnett, back to Beall, and now back to Barnett was very confusing. The entire ordeal quickly became a blur to me, and I just went through the motions as best I could. I was relieved that testing had ruled out a brain tumor and multiple sclerosis, but remained alarmed because my condition continued to worsen. I was unaware of the overall general pattern of the progression or stabilization of my symptoms. During sleep, the problems were gone, but these hours of refuge were shattered always by the persistent symptoms that greeted me faithfully every morning. Dr. Harch later explained that dealing with those symptoms every morning with disappointment was classic for brain injury, because brain injuries don't just go away.

I continued to be plagued by fears of being abandoned. It was quite evident that some of my family showed less support for me, especially when it came to my emotional pain. Some relatives too quickly attributed my problems to a "merely" psychological origin. Their words cut deeply. "Dan, you'd better get a hold of yourself" or "C'mon now, just pull yourself up by your bootstraps and get over this." Nothing is worse than a bunch of pretend psychologists attempting to solve a neurological problem with quaint, yet inadequate adages.

Of course, I am the first to admit that I was no angel during these trying times. Cursing, ranting, and raving were too often my only recourse, and I had many explosive fits of rage. My mood swings were incredible, and I attempted to pacify myself with meditation and prayer.

Before I experienced these problems, I didn't understand why people committed suicide. In truth, I thought them somewhat weak or inferior. But, continually harangued by neurological symptoms and compounding family strife, I went from accepting my limitations to seriously contemplating suicide. These symptoms were all the worse because they made me appear as though I had been drinking again.

Following the day of neurological testing, my mother drove me to the hyperbaric unit at the Regional Medical Center. The monoplace (meaning designed for one person) hyperbaric chamber was a long, clear cylinder positioned lengthwise. There were heavy, cast-iron or molded metal caps on both ends of the tube, and one end had a round door hanging on very large, smooth hinges. The clear tube was either made of acrylic, Plexiglas, or some other type of special glass. A cushioned stretcher fit on two parallel shiny metal rails that ran the length of the cylinder. I would spend two hours a day for the next three days in that tube.

I changed into a hospital gown, and after the hyperbaric technician listened to my heart and lungs, he checked my ears. He then explained how the treatment worked and assured me that everyone outside the chamber would be able to hear me, and I could hear them when they spoke into a special microphone. As I learned about the process, my fears were replaced with glorious hope.

As the air hissed with a sound like a pressure cooker into the chamber, I lay on my back and stared through the clear acrylic glass at a mobile of plastic hang gliders that dangled from the room's ceiling. My first adventure with hyperbaric medicine had begun.

4
MORE SETBACKS

Hyperbaric oxygen therapy—known as HBOT—is a treatment like none other. On one hand, it looks elaborate and forbidding, on the other hand its concept is quite straightforward. So with attendants close by with whom I could communicate through a special microphone, I felt reassured and relaxed. Lingering fear was replaced with glorious hope. Each day, before treatment began, the hyperbaric technician listened to my heart and lungs and checked my ears. (During treatment, air pressure in the middle ear is balanced with the increasing pressure inside the chamber.) The technicians also explained that improved vision is often an unexpected benefit of HBOT. While this information had no relevance to me at the time since I didn't wear glasses, it stuck with me and seemed rather peculiar. Was hyperbaric oxygen really capable of such magic? Perhaps so.

The only magic I hoped for was a return of my balance. At that time, I still didn't fully realize just how profoundly my thought processes had been affected. It seemed that all I could focus on was my balance and ability to walk, almost completely forgetting that I could no longer play the piano or guitar, and I couldn't operate a computer keyboard.

I felt distracted when the technician asked me which TV channel I wanted to watch. I didn't care, because I tried to concentrate only on the cure I knew would soon occur. It is strange to look back and realize that I thought I could concentrate my way into recovery, even though my thought processes were so out of whack. But my hope was strong—against all odds. I prayed for a miracle. I wasn't about to give up just yet.

The air hissed into the chamber. The plan was to start with 1.5 atmospheres for a specific amount of time, and then I would be placed under 2 atmospheres of pressure. Dr. Harch later explained to me that I was actually put at 2.8 atmospheres absolute, which is 1.8 times atmospheric pressure, adjusting for the New Mexico altitude. The sensation I experienced at 1.5 atmospheres was not unlike the feeling of being stretched out on my couch at home, but 2 atmospheres was different. I could definitely feel pressure on my entire body.

During treatment I lay on my back and stared at a mobile of brightly colored plastic hang gliders and their pilots that dangled from the ceiling. My mind drifted back to a friend from high school who had almost died in a hang gliding accident. Many people had prayed for him, and I wondered if the people in the church were praying for me now.

Over the one and a half hours I was in the chamber, the pressure was lowered back to 1 atmosphere, and the hissing sound returned. By the end of the treatment, I felt eager to get off of my back and try walking again, hoping that I could do it without being out of balance.

The hissing stopped after I was returned to normal atmospheric pressure. The technician opened the door with a sudden pop as if a seal were broken loose on a champagne bottle. He then pulled the white linen-wrapped bed out on the shiny parallel bars and told me to sit up slowly on the edge of the bed. After listening to my heart and lungs and examining my ears for pressure trauma, he told me to try walking. My heart jumped to my throat as my pulse began to race. I was both afraid and eager to try.

Carefully sliding off the monoplace bed, I tried to walk. No change! My heart sank. But I held on to hope. Maybe after tomorrow's treatment, I would be better. The technician cracked some kind of joke, but I wasn't able to appreciate his attempt at humor. But, lack of humor had plagued me throughout my long ordeal. I failed to remember jokes, much less understand the many jokes my extended family habitually bounced around.

This same routine went on for the next two days, and each day my hopes were dashed. By the end of the third treatment, I was very upset because I saw no change. In between treatments, during the days and evenings, I walked around my cousin Robbie's neighborhood, hoping that by practicing, my walking would improve. No difference. I still had to constantly struggle to stay in balance.

Those three days are etched into my memory, although all my memories are limited by my brain-damaged viewpoint during this phase of my life. I do recall the hot summer sun blazing down on the asphalt streets and concrete curbs of the lovely homes in my cousin's suburban community. I continued to struggle down the street, concentrating on placing one foot in front of the other while sweat poured from my brow, because I believed the hyperbaric oxygen treatments had failed—I was on my own again.

One minute I hoped these walking exercises might help, and the next minute I would be firmly convinced I was wasting my time. Sometimes, my thoughts centered on how many miles I'd need to walk in order to achieve balance again. Would I be able to walk straight after practicing one hundred miles? Would one thousand miles be sufficient? What about ten thousand miles? Okay, one hundred thousand miles? But then it would dawn on me that even if I practiced walking for a million miles, my balance would never return. Hopelessness settled in once again.

One hot afternoon, I rode along with Robbie, her husband, Bob, and the kids down to the country club. The kids and I headed for the swimming pool, while Robbie suntanned and Bob went out to play a round of golf. I tried to swim in the pool, but my disorientation issues became more apparent. I swam from one side of the pool to the other, but I always wound up off course.

I felt out of place in the pool with the kids. The "real" men were out playing golf, and so many attractive women were sunbathing. Usually, I was oblivious to my surroundings, but I began to hope that the water in the pool could heal me. Maybe, when I got out of the pool all of my problems would be washed away and I would walk normally again! Is it true that the pools of country clubs contain holy water with secret curative powers? Such were the thin and blurry lines that separated reality from wishful thinking.

The experience in the pool made me painfully aware of the fact that I no longer fit in with the "beautiful people" of the world. I was merely the handicapped visitor at the country club, doomed to never belong.

After the three HBOT treatments, considered experimental in the first place, the doctors decided to discontinue them. My experience with the treatments was surrealistic, and I remember little. Even now, I often wonder if they really happened.

Only much later would I learn about delayed hyperbaric oxygen therapy for decompression illness and the need for numerous HBOT treatments before success could be measured. I would have been in a state of disbelief had someone told me it would require eighty hyperbaric sessions in order for progress to be achieved. But, of course, I would have gladly participated in such therapy.

At that time, my father discussed the possibility of numerous delayed hyperbaric treatments with Dr. Schiller, who was the head of the Albuquerque HBOT unit, but he was rather cool about the idea. Apparently, he was unaware or arrogantly incapable of accepting such medical notions. At any rate, when my father mentioned Dr. Paul Harch's name and the proposed numerous hyperbaric treatments, Dr. Schiller simply dismissed Harch as nothing more than a charlatan or snake oil salesman. "Oh that guy," Dr. Schiller said. "Yes we have heard of him. But who in the world would want to have that many hyperbaric treatments?"

Although Dr. Harch talked to the doctors in New Mexico, he wasn't recommending my going to New Orleans for treatment and he didn't stand to profit from my case. Yet they still called him a charlatan and "just crazy."

Having numerous hyperbaric treatments is not an outlandish notion. HBOT is a noninvasive, painless treatment with few if any side effects. Certainly, it's true that desperate patients may be vulnerable to charlatans and quacks, but then, true innovators are often scorned initially and called crazy quacks. It's the way of the world. I often wonder what Dr. Schiller's skepticism was based on. Whatever it was, I know his judgment was distorted. That was the last I ever saw of him.

In one of my books about recovery from alcoholism, I found a quote about skepticism attributed to the philosopher, Herbert Spencer: *There is a principle which is a bar against all information, which is proof against all arguments and which cannot fail to keep a man in everlasting ignorance— that principle is contempt prior to investigation.*

I now wonder how any medical professional can so easily discount a reported treatment to a bewildered patient and send him or her on the way without any further hope or positive prognosis. How is it that our medical schools develop such doctors who perpetuate the everlasting ignorance because of a lack of any true investigation into the matter at hand?

During this time, my mother usually came with me to my medical consultations. Since I was unable to retain important information, she took notes and asked questions. Like many ill people, I was unable to advocate for myself. Fortunately, my two loving parents were willing to do it for me. My father continued searching for answers, often saying, "Surely, if we have the technology to send a man to the moon, there is a treatment for my son." Like my mother, he never gave up.

After the three HBOT treatments, I had no choice but to return home. At first, I insisted on driving and probably secretly hoped that the three treatments had improved my driving abilities. But not ten minutes north of the Albuquerque I became extremely frustrated and reacted physically, even tearing the turn signal from its steering wheel column, all the while cursing, ranting, and raving. Not a pretty sight.

My patient mother took over the driving and we continued the four-hour journey home. My mother has somehow found the patience to raise two difficult boys and be supportive of my father, too. She had also gone through the sudden death of her father and her mother's lengthy illness; taking her into our home during the last year of her mother's life. This remarkable woman also returned to school later in life to become a public elementary school teacher, and she spent twenty-three years teaching fifth grade.

While she attempted to care for me and believe in the possibility that I could be helped, she coped with unsupportive relatives who suggested I was mentally ill. This troubled her because she continued to believe that my problems resulted from the scuba diving incident at Lake Powell. Naturally, my fits of anger and rage wore on her. That day in the truck was no exception. After we arrived at my home that evening, she called my father and brother to come and help her deal with me. My mother's desperation was so apparent that they started the 400 mile drive immediately, arriving at my home an hour or so after the sun had risen over the bluffs in the canyon. I remember seeing my brother come into the den where I was sitting in a chair with all the life of a sack of potatoes. I stared blankly around the room and occasionally looked out the window to the top of the bluffs.

Lately, I'd been thinking irrational thoughts, such as, "If only I could get up to the top of the bluffs and muster the courage to jump to my death, I could solve my problems." Psychiatrists call this line of thinking "suicidal ideation." These destructive thoughts are not unusual for those who can find nothing about which to be hopeful. My life was no longer my own, and it was out of my control. I continually talked about killing myself—which made my loyal mother feel even worse. It's odd, too, that as much as I thought about killing myself, I was not about to take a drink! Suicide was now a possibility, but drinking could not even be considered.

My suicidal talk upset Ross, my brother, because of the negative effect it had on our mother. At one point, I wouldn't quit talking about suicide and we ended up in a physical fight. I remember trying to defend myself but losing handily to my younger and much stronger sibling. Later, with my brother sitting with me in silence, I resolved to keep my plans for suicide to myself and not upset my family with all that talk. I still planned to do it, though.

Dad wanted to take Mom home and leave Ross with me. My brother and I stayed silent in the den while they talked in another room. I continued to stare into space, saddened by my mental condition, yet powerless to do anything about it. At that time, the brain damage dampened my emotions, and I experienced sadness more as an uncomfortable feeling rather than true sadness. The same was true with joy. The only day I felt somewhat joyous would have been on the return trip from my initial appointment with Dr. Barnett, when I found out that I did not have a brain tumor or multiple sclerosis. But even then, the emotion was not felt as joy, rather it was the awareness of a good thing rather than a bad thing.

I could feel and correctly identify anger, but I likely experienced it much like a wounded animal would—all defenses were up, and I couldn't consider the presence or feelings of others. I pounded my fists into walls and stomped on the floor, in angry defiance of my balance problems and gait dysfunction. Sometimes, I pounded my fists into the keyboard of my studio piano in the vain attempt to find the correct keys in order to play simple childhood songs. Still, in all its fiery power, anger was the only true emotion I could experience, and it made me feel close to normal.

The realization that I was driving my mother away snapped me back into the hard reality of my situation. Consequently, I chose silence. The world was passing me by, and there seemed to be nothing I could do about it. All the doctors and well-intentioned family members could no longer help me. Should I indeed dash myself on the boulders at the base of the sandstone bluffs? They were the same bluffs upon which I not so long ago sat and watched the sunset and contemplated serenity, sobriety, the connections of mortality with immortality, and the very meaning of life.

When my parents came into the room, I saw that my mother's makeup was smeared on her cheeks. She had suffered so.

"You have got to promise me that you are going to be okay," she said.

I attempted to nod to assure her that I'd be all right. I even believed that a little.

She told me she and my dad were leaving. I looked at her, but my neck was frozen in a stiff posture and I couldn't nod or turn my head.

She asked again if I'd be okay, and I managed to mumble some sort of affirmative answer.

My dad then reverted to an old joke that he had told a million times when we were growing up. "You know what George Washington told his men before they crossed the Delaware?" We'd all play along and look blank, but then he'd say, "Get in the boat!"

I listened with one ear. I'd heard the joke a million times before, and I knew it was Dad's way to remind us to keep things simple and basic. I tried to nod and attempted a smile. By this time, I looked forward to the break from my mother, as if her absence might improve my mental outlook. I continually played the mental card in my head that told me I'd be okay if I could just get away from home, or I'd be okay if I could just go back home. Maybe I'd be okay if Mom would leave, or then again, maybe it was better that she stay.

My parents left the next morning, much to my relief, knowing that they were escaping this living hell. I resolved not to let Mom down, no matter how depressed I might become.

My brother Ross, a friendly, fun loving man with a great sense of humor, stayed behind. Ross had been through quite a few trials in life himself, including, at age twenty-five, heart surgery for the replacement of a heart valve. I had always admired his common sense approach to life, and I respected how courageous he had remained through all of his ordeals. I believed his presence would be refreshing.

That day, I tried to read short stories from one of my Alfred Hitchcock mystery magazines, but reading was such a struggle, I ended up sleeping more than usual. I stayed away from challenging things for fear of losing my temper. Besides, my hands were already bruised from pounding the keyboard and the walls. I was afraid of driving Ross away.

The next day, we had an appointment with the neurologist. Ross got ready to go and coaxed me to get into the freshly cleaned truck.

Just before pulling out of the driveway, Ross turned to me and said, "You want me to take you to that doctor in New Orleans? I can drive you there."

"No," I said. I couldn't even remember the doctor's name. By this time, I figured he would be one more doctor who couldn't help me. I could still hear the voice of Dr. Schiller warning my father about the quackery of some doctor in Louisiana. At the time, I didn't know any better, so I envisioned some shifty-eyed snake oil salesman in a shack in the steamy southern swamps.

I resigned myself to another trip to see Dr. Barnett, halfway across the state. All I knew was that the three hyperbaric treatments had not changed a thing in my condition.

That evening we stayed with my cousin, Robbie, and watched movies on the VCR. I began to see that if I could just sit quietly and watch the movie, nothing more would be required of me. Perhaps watching movies could be my new pastime. I wouldn't have to talk or even laugh at the humorous parts. No one discussed the plots of the various movies either. So, for the brief time I stayed with Robbie, I quietly accepted my newfound existence in the world of movies.

5

BRAIN DAMAGE

Many times I had trouble focusing on information I was given about my condition. I had fallen into a numb state of mind and had let go of expectations. For example, at my next appointment with Dr. Barnett, he said something about making an appointment with a neuropsychologist to determine the extent of the brain damage. Did he say "brain damage?" I had thought the MRI, and all the other testing to which I'd been subjected, had revealed no abnormalities. From that point on, I didn't hear anything past "brain damage." Not that it mattered much, because Dr. Barnett talked more directly to my brother than he did me.

I had reached a place within the profile of disability in which I no longer was treated as my own advocate, and therefore I was not dealt with directly. I know many others have been in similar situations; one in which we feel as if we are reduced to the status of heavy cargo. In my case, my brother became responsible for carting me around. I'm sure many other people can relate, because many families must cope with varying degrees of disability and disabling disease.

"Did he say brain damage?" I asked Ross—several times—as we walked back to the truck.

"Yes, he did, Dan," Ross replied in his typical Western twang.

Everything went into slow motion. Even though the symptoms persisted, I had never heard a diagnosis. While I'd found that maddening, the words "brain damage" didn't sit well either. And what did that mean exactly? What difference would the label make? At that point, I wasn't sure. I'd been relieved to know that my symptoms didn't result from a brain tumor, multiple sclerosis, or some other life-threatening malady. Despite the plethora of armchair diagnoses and therapy coming from various family members, I never bought into the idea that my symptoms were purely emotional or psychological, or in other words, mental illness. I knew deep in my heart that there was more to this than simplistic psychological mumbo jumbo.

For me, decompression sickness sounded less threatening than "brain damage." Still, I felt some relief to at long last hear a diagnostic term used and have an appointment with new specialists. Having already been through so much emotional turmoil over my condition, I was no longer afraid. Over the years, I've discovered that we humans can only take so much stress, and at some point, additional stress has little effect.

Later that day, I watched everyone around the table at Robbie's house drinking a beer or a glass of wine with our dinner. It dawned on me that these individuals could drink all evening, and they'd never mess up their brain as badly as mine was messed up. It was unfair. I'd spent so much time sobering up, yet I was the one with the slurred speech and the short-term memory deficits. But my sobriety was critical to me. I'd quit my position as the administrator of the night school and my teaching career was in jeopardy, so I had nothing else to hang on to but my sobriety. To pick up the first beer or first glass of wine would mean throwing away what little chance I had of surviving. I prayed the Serenity Prayer so many times that I thought I might wear it out.

One night after dinner, I went for a walk—or rather, I hobbled around the neighborhood, staying as close to the curb as possible to avoid falling into the traffic. As I wandered, I thought about what my future might hold. Maybe I could change my name and move to Roswell, New Mexico (don't ask me why), and become a janitor at a school. I would sell my musical instruments and buy a nice VCR to watch endless hours of movies during my time off and on weekends. Once I changed my name, I would be free to be "brain damaged Dan," no longer needing to impress anyone. In time, I could forget the person I'd been, the Dan with dreams and aspirations that could never again exist. I'd remove myself from friends and family, too.

The next morning, Robbie drove me across the river into Albuquerque for my appointment with the neuropsychologists. While in the waiting room, I picked up a popular magazine with Michael Landon's picture on the cover. Sadly, he had recently died from pancreatic cancer, and the article said something about his final triumphant struggle with death. I got that general impression, although I lacked the ability to focus on or remember anything I read. The cover picture showed him when he was younger and in much better health, and I couldn't help but feel sad that "Little Joe" was no longer with us.

That train of thought led me to think of Landon's heroic struggle. Rather than being inspired by it, I ended up feeling sad, knowing that in my current struggles I would never be heroic like Landon. I feared I lacked that heroic spirit and didn't have that same courageous fiber. In fact, I'd scared off people in my family with my ranting and raving and acting like a madman. But that morning, I felt fairly rested as I worked to accept that I was truly brain damaged. In my typical fashion, I was also curious about the upcoming testing. I even began to think of it as a welcomed change.

That morning, when I had my initial appointment with Dr. Curley, he asked many questions about the scuba diving incident at Lake Powell. Obviously, this was a story I had told dozens—hundreds!—of times. At the conclusion of the interview, he shared his doubts that I actually had decompression illness. His reaction didn't upset me too much. After all, most of the professional people I had met thus far had expressed similar doubts.

The testing came next, although a different person actually administered these tests, which consisted of question-answer segments, memory tests involving numbers, and sorting cards. At one point I was blindfolded and asked to put together some puzzle pieces of different shapes using touch only. I also copied designs and later reproduced them from memory. I was in trouble on many of the memory tests—I didn't need a Ph.D to tell me that. Yet, I couldn't help but hope that I was performing well for the woman administering the test—I found her attractive and that fed the desire to do well.

Robbie arrived to take me to lunch, which presented another challenge. I'd gained weight since my accident, and since I walked at such a slow pace, I'd lost much of my former fitness. Although eating was a tiring experience, I still looked forward to meals. My accident had left me with difficulties with food, and with each bite I had to be careful not to choke. No matter how careful I tried to be, I always ended up spilling something on my shirt, and when that happened, I reacted badly. At lunch that day, Robbie tried to soothe me and tell me not to be so hard on myself. Easy for her to say. She wasn't spilling food into her lap or struggling just to sip from a glass. I was embarrassed every day. Fortunately, I could remember who I had been and what I had accomplished and hung on to the hope that I could resurrect the old Dan.

I spent the rest of the day trying to do well on more tests. Since the examiner was so attractive and I'd become taken with her smile, I was even more eager to do well and impress her. The pressure was on! After a couple of hours of tests that measured various abilities from verbal to numerical to spatial skills, we moved on to testing that involved emotional and psychological probing. This was not my favorite portion, because I became confused as to how to answer them. Should I respond from the perspective of the old Dan before the scuba diving incident or from the perspective of the new, brain damaged Dan? The fact that my short-term memory abilities were not up to par didn't help either. In addition, I had trouble manipulating the pencil and using the correct pressure within the confines of the "bubbled" answer sheet. The process was exhausting.

The next day, I had yet another medical appointment, this one with a leading ear, nose, and throat specialist in the state. This was to determine if my balance problems might be related to some inner ear damage or an ear infection. Mom, Dad, and Rita, Ross' musically talented girlfriend, drove across the state to meet us. That afternoon, my mother and I drove over for the appointment with Dr. Thorne. The testing included an ENG exam, because he explained that I might have an inner ear fistula that could cause balance problems. After the test, he said he wanted to see me again in two weeks. What was it with doctors and this two-week thing? However, in this case, I was relieved that we were going to wait two weeks before considering surgery. While surgery to patch up a possible fistula might improve my balance problems, he also said that the fistulas usually corrected themselves with time.

After that appointment, we drove back across the state. Ross and Rita rode in my GMC pickup truck, while I rode with Mom and Dad. The trip was very tiring, made worse by my ruminations about the possibility I'd be facing surgery. Dr. Thorne's description of the surgery was enough to make me desperately want this balance issue to resolve on its own. I even considered lying about feeling better in order to avoid the surgery. So, after all, maybe I wasn't willing to do *anything* to cure my balance problems.

My parents stayed painfully quiet about the diagnosis of brain damage. Maybe they were doing so to avoid the tragic realization that something indeed had happened to me that might not be fixable. I stayed at my parents' house for the next thirteen days and spent my time sleeping and watching movies with Rita and Ross, but also walking as much as possible. About this time I started practicing to improve my handwriting. I'd noticed that I made mistakes in forming letters and also omitting letters within words. It seemed, though, that these small neurological glitches continued no matter how much I practiced writing on that yellow pad.

I attempted to comfort myself by making comparisons with other situations. I'd say that I wasn't suffering like my grandmother had during her final weeks of coping with cancer. As much as I tried, these thoughts felt shallow and I never found true peace in my meditations. Despite this, my spiritual path was working, because I maintained my sobriety, and I hadn't started smoking either. It would have been easy because Ross and Rita smoked while we watched movies on the VCR every evening. But that would have been a disaster. With my memory deficits I would have left burning cigarettes all over the place.

Visits with my friend Lee Ann were important because she was spiritually strong and truly had the faith of a mustard seed. We had been high school classmates who, years later, developed a spiritual connection by telephone, following her divorce and me sobering up. I welcomed her encouragement as a bright ray of optimism, even though I thought she was just whistling in the dark. Facts are facts, and wishful thinking is just wishful thinking. But I didn't argue with Lee Ann, not that I could have argued even if I'd wanted to, since my mental abilities weren't up to sparring with others. But Lee Ann had opened her home and shared what she had, even though she was living modestly with her three children at the time.

We often prayed together and read from the Bible, and even in my reduced mental capacity, she didn't treat me like a handicapped person. I never scoffed to her face about her staunch belief that I would be healed, but I remained skeptical. On the practical side, she also helped me find nutritional and herbal remedies. Lee Ann would become a crucial link to God for me in the next few months.

Back when things were going great in my life, I had bought two sculpture pieces to give to my parents for Christmas. Both sculptures sat on the television console, and I would often look up at them when I would awaken from my frequent daytime naps. One piece was of a victorious Native American performing the powerful "Eagle Dance." Although I didn't understand all the meaning behind this piece, it conveyed a sense of victory and freedom. The other piece was that of a Native American with his head held down, sitting on his emaciated horse. I believe it was called the "End of the Trail" and captured despair and defeat in the human spirit. Those two pieces symbolized the contrast in my life. I had once felt like the spirit of the powerful eagle dancer, but now I was like the man at the end of the trail.

While I waited for my next doctor's appointments, I visited a local nursing home where I had worked as an orderly while putting myself though college. I went in an effort to cheer myself up by seeing a young man there named Ray, who had a severe case of cerebral palsy. His left side was drawn up, and he had limited use of his right hand. At first glance, Ray was a rather scary sight, but that changed once anyone got to know him. His smile brightened the darkest room in the nursing home, even though he couldn't talk. Ray spent most of the day strapped into a padded wheelchair and could only make three hand signals—a closed fist for "no," an okay sign for "yes", and he could flip people off when he was angry. Oh yes, he could also motion a finger toward his nostril in order to convey the meaning of "up your nose." While working as an orderly, I was told that Ray could not control his arms; however, he traditionally broke in the new orderlies when he was upset by hitting them in the groin. Ouch! That Ray could pack a punch.

I had begun to develop a communication board for Ray, and he had really been catching on. However, not many workers in the nursing home were willing to use the tool, so Ray was trapped in a slow but effective binary system of yes and no hand signals in order to effectively communicate with others.

I visited Ray with the hope of feeling grateful for my own life. Why was I contemplating suicide when I was lucky enough to be able to speak? Ray had never spoken a word in his life. I chastised myself for my lack of gratitude. I told Ray about my accident and asked him to pray for me. He assured me that he would, and I left feeling encouraged. I never saw Ray again, and I later learned that he had died after a bout with cancer.

I sometimes think about Ray, who couldn't speak, and can't help but think about how often I kept myself from speaking. For example, if I used the term "brain damage," my parents would become upset and ask me not to use those words. On the other hand, Robbie liked to make odd jokes about everyone having "drain bamage."

Meanwhile, fear gripped my soul. I still imagined my brain being occupied by some hideous woolly spider crouching on eight legs somewhere in the corner of my skull, slowly devouring the soft tissues of my brain. With every new morning, I awakened to the possibility of decreasing cognitive abilities.

During this time, a girl named Gina became my inspiration. To this day, I honor Gina who had been in my mother's fifth-grade class. At the time I was ill, Gina was battling leukemia and not expected to live. Gina became like a guardian angel to me. How well I remember stumbling down the street to visit her. I hadn't seen her since she was a toddler, and now she was an elementary student without a future. Staying in my parents' home down the street from Gina, it was easy to remember her. However, it was difficult to do so when I had a most troublesome time remembering anyone who was literally out of sight. My memory was dominated by an out of sight, out of mind predicament. While waiting with my parents in my hometown of Portales, there were minutes during the days that I could remind myself of Gina and feel gratitude for my own life. Away from that environment, I had trouble remembering her. For those precious moments when I was with Gina, she helped me from descending into a depression that would suck my soul even deeper into the watery grave of my consciousness—a description that kept coming back to me, and for a reason.

When I was in the eleventh grade, I once experienced a vision that seemed to come from nowhere. It happened while I sat idly in the last ten minutes of chemistry class, as other students fed mice to the rattlesnake that the biology teacher kept. The only way to describe what came next is to say that suddenly, my consciousness flew from the room, and I began writing on a white sheet of notebook paper. I wasn't consciously thinking these words, but rather, they seem to spring from deep within. I've never been able to reference my words in any known source. Later, I submitted this piece to the Eastern New Mexico University's literary magazine *El Portal*. I'm reproducing it here to close out this chapter for reasons that will become obvious when you read it.

REALITY?

The dark water was all around me. It was over, under, and in every direction I could see. My tortured soul screamed for life, as tons of pressure gagged the last molecules of air from my recalcitrant lungs. Catching a faint glimmer of hope out of the corner of my slowly closing eyes, I saw the surface—that interface which meant the difference between life and death. I pushed upward hard and fast to find myself tossed upon the heaving waves of an angry sea. Once again I almost gave up hope, when suddenly out of the stormy skies flew a gigantic bird such as I had never seen before—a gigantic, brilliant-white albatross. It flew straight toward me, picked up my weakened body, and I was carried high above the watery jaws of death.

It felt so good to be high above my ultimate doom. The giant bird then flew toward sun-drenched seas with a surface as smooth as glass. I then was placed upon a sandy beach—a long, clean, brilliant-white sandy beach which stretched infinitely into the horizons. After a long rest and an attempt to regain my breath, I picked my weary form up and began to walk along the white shore. Looking to my left, I saw the endless universe of liquid blue; however, to my right was the jungle. It was thick and green—a solid wall of flora, impenetrable. Varieties of brilliantly colored fruits clung to vines and branches. Suddenly, I was overcome by the many colors which the convolutions of my brain could not understand. The reds, oranges, sun-yellows, the dark wall of jungle, the deep-blue sea, the light blue, the glaring sun . . . but worst of all was the endless brilliant white sand which stretched to infinity. I was filled with hysteria . . . I ran wildly . . . aimlessly . . . down the beach until all the colors blended into a brilliant white sand which surrounded me at first . . . then mysteriously came to life. The sand jumped at my eyes, stinging them with such pain that I could hardly keep them open. Then the sharp particles of brilliant white angrily jumped at my nostrils and mouth as if to stifle my very breath. With the sand filling every pore of my skin and my apertures for breath, I convulsed in one last effort to resist death; I quickly found that it was much easier just to give in . . .

So I relaxed . . . and the albatross flew toward me with his eyes red with hatred—that kind of life-killing hatred. He clenched me by the neck and quickly flew me to where I belonged . . . a body . . . slowly sinking toward the bottom . . . the white-sanded bottom of a tempest-tossed sea.

6
THE ONGOING TAILSPIN

A sad event occurred during the two weeks I stayed with my parents and waited for my second appointment with Dr. Thorne. Glen, an old friend of mine, had fallen asleep while smoking a cigarette and died in the fire that started as a result. Some years back, Glen and I had worked at the nursing home together. He'd taught me much about caring for the elderly and severely handicapped people and had introduced me to Ray, the young man with cerebral palsy. Glen was also a musician and played a beautifully crafted twelve-string guitar, while I clunked along on my cheap six-string guitar—both of us making up words as we went along.

Glen and I had been friends for the past ten years and stayed in touch even after I moved far away. An extremely intelligent man, he was interested in philosophy and metaphysics, and at one point he decided that saving money to buy a telescope in order to closely monitor Halley's Comet as it returned to our solar system was more important than buying a much needed car. He continued to ride his bike everywhere so that he could afford his prized telescope.

The news of Glen's sudden and tragic death sent me into a tailspin. I couldn't even muster the fortitude to attend his funeral, and I couldn't even cry for him. It seemed that my ability to cry was gone forever, although I was despondent over the loss of Glen.

Looking back, it's a wonder to me that my family loved me enough to put up with my incredible mood swings and outbursts during these long periods of waiting and the frustration that went along with them. But each day my mother encouraged me to walk, attempt to play the piano, and practice writing on the yellow notepad. For his part, my father encouraged me to have faith that the medical doctors would eventually help me. Meanwhile, my brother provided me with comic relief when we watched movies at his house. From time to time, I would visit with Lee Ann, who also encouraged me to continue to believe that God would do marvelous things, even when I lost faith. Still, at times I felt certain that my life was over.

One Sunday, Rita, Ross, and I were asked to sing together at the First Baptist Church for the senior adult class. Rita was studying to become a music therapist, and she played the guitar to accompany her lovely voice. Although I could no longer sing too well, Dad encouraged me to go along with Rita and Ross. This was a daunting undertaking. The problems with my memory were significant, and the strength of my voice had changed, too, so it was softer than it had been before. In addition, I had less control over annunciation and breathing. On the other hand, at one time I'd sung in the bars and nightclubs to pick up extra money, so maybe I hadn't been too bad.

I had to face the fear of looking foolish in front of others, but I went to church anyway. Dressed in a suit and tie, I sweated in the July heat, and I wasn't happy with my father for more or less making me do this—I felt like the organ grinder's monkey.

The kind of mental shape I was in didn't change for occasions like this. In other words, I couldn't rise to the occasion, because I didn't have the inner resources to draw on. For example, as we entered the church building, I asked a gray-haired woman where all the old folks were. I immediately knew I'd blurted out something that shouldn't be said aloud. The unfriendly way the woman pointed to the senior class made me even more aware that I'd misspoken.

So much for social graces. Sadly, I found that I blurted things that I normally would have kept to myself. My thoughts were almost transparent. Years later, Dr. Michael Shaughnessy explained that this behavior was termed "disinhibition." People who have suffered brain injury, particularly damage to the frontal lobe, often experience these problems and may cross lines from behavior that is considered appropriate into the realm of socially inappropriate words or actions.

That day, Rita and Ross did most of the singing, and I attempted to follow along. Of course, everyone was kind enough to let us think we were wonderful, but I knew that I was just the monkey with the two organ grinders. Ross and Rita sang well enough, and Rita's guitar playing was superb. As I saw it, however, I was the freak show portion of the entertainment. I was painfully aware of my deficits that persisted.

One afternoon, my mother and I went to the university library to research information about decompression illness, although I knew that this kind of "cognitive demand" would exhaust me for days. That day, I fumbled my way through the index of *The MERCK Manual*, a medical reference book. My eyes struggled with the material under the symptoms, signs, and diagnosis section. I had mixed feelings when I read that losing consciousness was a common symptom of decompression sickness, the "bends." That hadn't happened to me, nor had I experienced convulsions. Since I didn't understand what the line about "other CNS manifestations" meant, I passed over it and read on. All in all, based on what I read, it seemed possible that my symptoms weren't related to the diving incident at all.

I hadn't experienced the symptoms listed under "milder symptoms and signs" either. For the most part, I was again relieved that I didn't show symptoms of pulmonary damage. I had not found enough information from my diver-training manual to help me out, but I'd had a feeling that perhaps *The MERCK Manual* would hold the answer to my current condition. This was important to me because I'd begun to really resent the psychological explanations—too many untrained people, including family members, seemed all too eager to explain away my symptoms as a mental illness.

Unfortunately, that day's research gave me no comfort, but instead left me fearful of things to come. I stuck with *The MERCK Manual*, seeing it as a holy text of scientific truth about my condition. I spent the entire afternoon looking up things I didn't understand, learning that, of course, CNS meant "central nervous system." Reading further really opened my eyes, and the section on neurological manifestations indicated that "major cerebral problems" could be included. I certainly experienced cerebral—and not "emotional"—problems. Among the facts that enlightened me was a notation that the vertigo associated with decompression illness was difficult to differentiate from the inner ear fistula, for which Dr. Thorne was currently monitoring me. Finally! An explanation for the balance problems.

In that one clear moment, I no longer doubted that I had decompression illness. My relief didn't last long because as I read on I learned that "bone necrosis," dying bone tissue, was sometimes detected months or years after the event that caused it. Worse, a single improper decompression could cause this condition.

I went numb with fear. As if I didn't have enough to worry about. Now, rotting bones? Was that why I couldn't walk normally, but showed an unsteady gait? My thoughts drifted back to an old Rod Sterling *Night Gallery* episode in which the main character was injected with medicine that was going to turn him into a slimy, spineless, worm. The character found a gun and shot himself rather than face the outcome of becoming a worm.

I left the library enraged by what I believed I'd done to myself. That was my perception. I blamed myself for not identifying the decompression event and seeking help immediately. Although I had found the correct diagnosis, I could find no hope in my prognosis. I slapped the notepad against the walls of the library and thrashed the notebook through some shrubs as I staggered out to the car to await my mother to drive me back home. I made a scene, showing my rage for the few college students passing nearby.

"Well, I have decompression illness," I told my mother.

"We need to visit with Dr. Thorne," she replied.

"That inner ear balance stuff is a bunch of crap."

"Let's see what the doctors say, dear," she said, in a reassuring tone.

I began to cry softly—my ability to cry had returned. In my mind, I visited to Lake Powell and replayed the event, this time imagining myself avoiding the uncontrolled ascent. I ended up with self-blame yet again, asking God why I had done this to myself. Worse, I now had medical terms in my head. Osteonecrosis! When would my bones rot and die? By the time my imagination had worn itself out, I saw myself as bedridden, completely helpless. And why not? Clearly, my condition had not improved no matter how many miles I walked or how many times I practiced writing on my yellow pad. The thought of killing myself began to take root. Fortunately, I had no definite plan.

As I descended into this mental hell, my father insisted that I did not have brain damage—he got angry whenever I mentioned the possibility. Meanwhile, my mother continued to encourage me to practice writing and walking.

Although my parents talked in encouraging terms, they'd become so concerned about my increasing despondency and talk of suicide that they made an appointment for all of us to visit with a long-time family friend and doctor, Dr. Robert Timmons. My parents were comfortable with this doctor, who showed a great deal of common sense and wisdom. I don't remember much about the visit, and Dr. Timmons didn't have any additional medical information, but in front of my parents, he told me that killing myself would be a terrible waste of a human life. His wisdom was like a small light breaking through the clouds of depression, however briefly.

Finally, my parents drove me two hundred miles across the state to Albuquerque for the appointment with Dr. Curley, the neuropsychologist to whom I had been referred by Dr. Barnett, for the results of my neuropsychological testing and to find out the nature of my brain damage. We'd also see Dr. Thorne, but I'd already made up my mind that I was not going to undergo surgery for an inner ear problem I no longer believed I had.

The meeting with Dr. Curley shocked me, because his recommendation was to learn to accept my condition—and attempt to practice the Serenity Prayer. This was all he could tell me? I could not believe my ears! I knew all about the battle to understand the difference between the things I could not change and the things I could. Dr. Curley's pleasant voice droned on with more gibberish about acceptance and something about emotional distress. He mentioned nothing about brain damage or decompression illness. Of course, I was relieved that his findings did not indicate "lateralized brain dysfunction." But neither could he tell me the extent of the brain damage. His final recommendation was for me to seek counseling.

My parents and I were in a state of disbelief, although my father attempted to focus on the positive aspects. In fact, Dr. Curley's interpretation of the evaluation results supported emotional distress. My average performance on the tests conducted by the attractive woman did not support the existence of a brain injury. During lunch, my mother appeared pleasant, while I continued to express my disbelief. I also hated to think about all the relatives who would gloat over the news that I showed no evidence of brain damage and that my problems were emotional. Oh, how I dreaded the "group therapy" session with my relatives that evening when we gathered for their happy hour with drinks and gossip.

Later, Dad drove us to Dr. Thorne's office, where my cousin Dee Ann, a personal friend of Dr. Thorne's, met us. Unfortunately, because of my bad feelings toward Dee Ann, her presence added to my growing mistrust. Not that it mattered. Dr. Thorne essentially said that time would heal my balance problems. With no other diagnosis offered to explain my symptoms, the "Dan is emotionally ill" crowd had their way! But because of what I'd read in *The MERCK Manual,* I was convinced that the inner ear issue was part of the decompression illness that I felt sure was the real diagnosis.

I drove home with Dee Ann—why that happened is beyond me. The gist of her line of talk was that "everything would be all right." I just needed counseling. I was infuriated at first, but soon I resigned myself to accept the ultimate escape. How hard could it be to kill myself? I kept silent but thought about suicide, while Dee Ann droned on.

Unfortunately, the underlying frustration and tension seethed with the power of a volcano. My cousin scolded me when I shared my fears that I would eventually take my own life. Her terse, sarcastic words taunt me even now. "Be sure to do it outside so that it won't be such a terrible mess for people to clean up." That kind of sarcasm was not helpful. Over the next period of time, graphic suicidal thoughts continued.

Although sleep provided relief from my thoughts and the humming conch shell in my ears, I'd awaken with horrible thoughts about a worsening condition—decaying bones and my mind unraveling at its own unpredictable rate. One day I might not even know my name or where I lived. My life had finally culminated at this point of complete desolation and profound depression.

We gathered in Robbie's lovely home for a big feast. But all I remember is that everyone expressed their great relief that all these doctors had found nothing wrong with me. The increasing cacophony created by all this odd celebration disturbed me greatly. At one point I mustered the strength to utter, "But why can't I play the piano anymore?"

My aunt Shirley quickly reminded me that I could still play the radio. Dee Ann jumped in with talk of a good psychotherapist she knew. Uncle R.T. added that he'd known that therapist for years.

"But I have decompression illness," I quietly interjected.

"You don't know what the hell you have, Dan!" Dee Ann yelled.

The whirlwind of armchair psychological mumbo jumbo was more than I could bear. I unsteadily stood up and walked to the door.

"Where are you going, sweetie?" Robbie asked.

"I am getting the hell out of here!" I screamed.

My parents left with me and we drove to the hotel, but they continued talking about the "medical events" of the day. As far as I could see, all I ended up with was a recommendation to seek counseling. At least I wasn't being urged to have surgery, and that left me greatly relieved.

Even without results that satisfied me, I'd learned in my twelve-step recovery program to be open-minded and willing to seek help. So, although I seriously contemplated suicide, I remained open to at least seeing a professional counselor to help me adjust to this situation. What choice did I have? I felt better when I left my "expert" family members and was alone with my parents, my brother, and his girlfriend, all of whom were my true sources of support.

I still believed that I had decompression illness, no matter what everyone else thought. My father also secretly believed it, because he'd begun to question the conclusions of experts, and instead, listened to Rita's mother, who happened to be a special licensed nurse/medical practitioner. Unbeknownst to me, sometime during all of this turmoil, Rita's mother sent Dad a photocopied set of papers regarding decompression illness.

How ironic that as I began to struggle to decide whether to continue my life, my father silently began his search for answers. As I began to give up, he started to fight my illness with everything he had. He would become my chief defender and silent supporter.

7
TRYING TO ACCEPT THE UNACCEPTABLE

The next day my mother and I went back to my house in Farmington, and my father returned to our hometown of Portales. My plan was to contact a psychologist to begin psychotherapy. No more hyperbaric treatments and no more medical doctor appointments. This was the plan, but I knew deep in my heart that I could sit around and talk about my problems until the end of time, but that wouldn't help me get back my balance and thinking abilities. By this time, I just wanted my brain back—I didn't care what it took.

Much twelve-step literature talks about acceptance, indicating that God has a purpose for everything, even the things we cannot accept. We can't find serenity until we accept our dilemmas and circumstances as exactly the way God has planned things. In many situations, this is sensible advice and truly is a path to serenity. It takes away resistance to seeing what is, rather than constantly fighting it. But I could not accept things the way they were.

Timothy, a good friend, came by one afternoon just as the sun was about to set. He urged me to go outside with him, so I managed to hobble out the door and follow him around the side of the house. He encouraged me to pay attention to the beautiful colors in the sky. True enough, the reds, oranges, and brilliant flame colors danced all over the few clouds of the desert dusk. The turquoise blues in the sky matched all too well the artistic temperament of the Native American earth over which they were suspended.

Tim used our time alone to encourage me to pull myself together and get on with my life. I could tell by his voice and his religious approach that even he no longer believed in a medical diagnosis. He, too, saw my problems as psychological and perhaps spiritual. All his advice would have been great if I'd had those problems. But I just wanted my brain back—my old brain, the one that worked, the one that played the piano and the guitar.

For the most part, my relatives and even the doctors had written me off as being crazy, although not all used the word openly. But over time, with so many people talking about me behind my back and even saying things that weren't true, support from professionals, family, and friends disappeared. At one point, a relative circulated the lie that in a fit of anger I'd thrown my mother to the ground. This was truly a lie, but knowing that others thought it was true sent me deeper into despair. Despite my belief in a physical cause of my symptoms, even I wondered if they were truly psychological—maybe I'd become schizophrenic.

Because of this kind of lie and other gossip, my parents and I gained insight into the family issues, and we began to stay in hotels on these medical trips. I've avoided certain family members ever since that troubling time.

I've talked with Dr. Harch about the way my physical and mental unraveling caused family ties to break. "The ties to *terra firma* were being severed," he said. We likened that to the oil platforms in the Gulf waters that have huge cables to anchor them and therefore help withstand heavy winds and ocean currents. Family is like the huge cables that anchored my abilities to stay rooted in reality. Eventually, though, they were severed one by one, and gradually I reached a point of breaking with reality.

As the days went on, I could not extricate myself from increasingly hopeless thoughts, including suicide. On the Sunday after I returned to my home in Farmington from visiting the Albuquerque doctors, I made my way back one last time to the church by the brook, where I had been attending during my early sobriety. Many loving Christians met me with open arms as I entered the sanctuary. Despite the welcome, I was sad that I could not have played music with the praise and worship team if my life depended on it.

My thought processes were so distorted that I felt guilty for wasting my life. I had not lived for the Lord, I thought. No, I had selfishly lived my life just for me. Unable to listen to the music or the message that day, I thumbed through my Bible, hoping for solutions for the problems that troubled my soul. I stopped at Psalm 69 where I managed to focus on the following words:

Save me, O God; for the waters are come in unto my soul. I sink in deep mire, where there is no standing: I am come into deep waters, where the floods overflow me. I am weary of my crying: my throat is dried: mine eyes fail while I wait for my God...O God, thou knowest my foolishness; and my sins are not hid from thee...I have become a stranger unto my brethren...They that sit at the gate speak against me; and I was the song of the drunkards...Deliver me out of the mire, and let me not sink: let me be delivered from them that hate me, and out of the deep waters. Let not the waterflood overflow me, neither let the deep swallow me up, and let not the pit shut her mouth upon me...And hide not thy face from thy servant; for I am in trouble: hear me..."

Somewhere during the end of that small Christian gathering, I began to weep quietly. The tears flowed down my cheeks. I knew that my situation was hopeless, and that I was directly responsible for inflicting my own wounds. I had become so deaf to God's plan in my life, that I was not able to hear Him attempting to stop me from that fateful dive that morning. My own selfish, demanding will had led me to my current brain damage. Such were my thought processes.

Several men and women gathered around me and placed their hands on me to pray. Soon, the whole group was gathered around me. Their faith was great, but mine was not. On top of that, I was ashamed that the only time I ran to God was when I needed something. I judged myself to be a horrible example of a Christian.

Despite my harsh judgments, I continued hoping that I'd wake each day cured—sound of body and mind. I would no longer weave and hobble as I walked. I'd have my mind back, too! Of course, that didn't happen, and each day my hopes were lost in fatigue and despondency.

What does a person do when there is no hope? All I could think of was the whitewashed gate in the backyard. I'd sit with my legs crossed in some sort of bizarre meditation pose just prior to sudden self-inflicted death. I imagined the bright sun beating down upon me as I sat there in my jeans, wearing my previously acquired diver's T-shirt, the one with a red diver's flag on it and the words that indicated that Sharon Smith had trained me. That T-shirt would be splattered with the blood of a dumb diver who had no idea of what the hell had happened to his life. It was all over. There was no possible way out of this hell scene. Death would be best.

I only had one problem. My mother was visiting me. She stayed at my house. I could not be rid of her. If only she would return across the state 400 miles away! Then I could in all good conscience hazardously drive out to the local Wal-Mart, and purchase the handgun I would need to complete my mission. I could not complete this mission with my mother at my house.

Finally, I gave up. There was no way I could get my mother to leave. I could not convince her that I would be all right if I were left alone. I stumbled into one of the empty bedrooms of my house and lay on the floor staring at the ceiling. Soon, I began crying uncontrollably. Eventually this led to a stream of obscenities and then a deluge of ravings. I was a madman trapped in his own body and brain and imprisoned in his own home.

I finally believed that I should shelve myself in some human warehouse for the remainder of my days. Locked away from the sunlight of civilization, and crouching in the dark corners of an insane asylum, I pictured myself no longer having to make any decisions, no longer having to function. I began to doubt every thought, every action, and even every breath I was taking. I couldn't walk or talk right. I couldn't play the piano anymore. I couldn't think. I couldn't live. I couldn't die. Now, I couldn't even kill myself, and I could not wait one more hour for any help.

Finally, my mother called Dr. Carroll, a well-known and respected Farmington psychiatrist whom she had heard about through her brother. Ironically, we never met this man nor received a bill from him. She was desperate to get help for me and to find some relief herself. He advised her to take me to the local medical center emergency room.

I was assured there were institutions for brain damaged individuals, and I wanted to go there, to be shelved.

"Are you sure that's what you want, Dan?" my mother asked several times.

My answer? "Yes, I just want to be shelved."

I silently sat in the passenger seat of the vehicle as she drove to the emergency room. I sought comfort in the fact that I had found the only possible answer to my problems. I had tried everything else and was down to my last option.

Once we were in the emergency room, a doctor gave me a physical exam, and, of course, found nothing wrong.

"I'm sorry that I embarrassed you with my life, Mom," I said after the doctor left. A strange calm acceptance enveloped my entire being. I was numb all over. Looking back on the troubled time, if I had been able to hear music in my brain I would have chosen Pink Floyd's "Comfortably Numb." But at the time, I had no music for my swan song, no dramatic background instrumentation for my farewell with my mother.

"I'm sorry that I let you down," I said.

I remember very little else about those final minutes with my mom in the emergency room examination room. I do not even recall Mom's exact words, but I'm sure she tried to comfort me and pray with me. By that time, though, I was being slowly enveloped in a silent, secret mental snow.

The doctor soon returned. "As you can see, we don't really have the facilities to help you here, Mr. Greathouse," he said.

"I just need to be shelved." I continued my mantra.

He turned his attention to my mother and ignored me. "We're making arrangements for you to take your son to the Sunrise Mental Health and Recovery Hospital. They are more equipped to deal with this type of case."

I heard the name of the Sunrise Mental Health and Recovery Hospital, but I didn't care that this was the place where I hadn't wanted to go. Not one hour earlier I was going to find a way to kill myself, so who was I to be picky?

Everything was a vague fog, but I do recall getting to the doors of Sunrise. Hell, I stumbled up to the place as if I owned it. It had not even been three years since I had been here the first time for alcoholism treatment. I felt at home in a strange sort of way. At least I would be getting away from the people and surroundings that would remind me of my painful losses.

"Are you sure this is what you want?" my mother asked.

"Yes!" I retorted, as I stormed on into the reception area to meet an intake person who had undoubtedly been tipped off about my arrival. I did not hug my mother, nor did I turn back to look at her. I completed the initial paperwork hoopla, which took an extraordinary amount of time. Then I saw an older nurse who remembered me from my previous stay.

"Did you slip and start drinking again?" she asked.

"No, I had a scuba diving accident. You have a *MERCK Manual*?" I asked.

Sure enough, there was a manual on the reference shelf. She pulled it down and handed it over to me. I showed her where it talked about osteonecrosis, and I explained to her that I no longer had a reason for living.

The same evening, Dr. Clifford Clairemont interviewed me in his office, but I didn't go into many details, as I was exhausted from telling my story to so many people who didn't believe me anyway.

"So, you wish to *off* yourself?" he calmly asked.

"Yes." I understood him to mean *off* as in kill myself.

"Do you have a plan?"

I went into elaborate detail about how I would obtain a gun, use a bag to avoid a mess, and blow my brains out. As I described this to him, I began wondering if I had not made a mistake coming back to Dr. Clairemont's hospital. Things just did not feel right here.

"Why did you come?" he asked.

"I just need to be shelved. I don't want to be rehabilitated or anything like that. I just want to be shelved."

"I can help you out, but you have to help me out while you're here," he talked seriously.

"Sure. What?" I asked.

"You have to promise not to *off* yourself while you're here on the ward," he said, looking at me with a serious expression.

"I promise I won't," I answered, thinking that it would be pretty much impossible to kill myself on the ward. Besides, I knew exactly where I was going to kill myself—the inside of my gate in the backyard. "I just need to be shelved," I repeated.

He smiled. "Don't worry, I can get you shelved. No problem."

With that, I was given a room to myself in the wing for chemically-dependent patients. In fact, it was right across the hallway from the room in which I had sobered up. All of the counselors were pleasant, and I recognized some of the same people I'd met three years earlier.

The next few days were simple, and the time was filled with meals, therapy groups, occupational therapy classes, and recreation time in the gym. I began a journal as written assignments were required as well. Although it took me much longer than the others to complete my work, I actively participated to the best of my ability. I didn't participate in hopes of recovering, or in hopes of improving my life. I was just passing the time as I waited to be permanently shelved. I figured it would be a couple of weeks before I'd be transferred to a permanent housing situation.

Each day began with the orderlies waking all psychiatric patients up at 7:00 AM, after which we had our vital signs checked and the meds were administered. Breakfast followed, and this facility offered way too much food. When I was there before, I gained weight, but this time, I struggled to keep from spilling food on myself at each meal. Then, after breakfast, we had a wake-up group therapy session, followed by recreation therapy, then two more, back-to-back, group therapy sessions before lunch, and two more after lunch. We had guided relaxation therapy sessions and then occupational therapy before dinner, followed by a lecture. Then we had two free hours and then another group therapy session before a snack and another free hour before lights out. The way I saw it, I'd be forced to survive a packed schedule of activities before I'd at last move on to a state institution, where I'd be without aim or purpose.

This hospital stay was nothing like I imagined. Somehow, these professionals thought my problems would be alleviated by so many group therapy sessions. I was amused at this approach, but not angry, because I considered it a mere bus stop along the path to the warehouse. All the psychotherapy in the world would not cure me.

This was my only alternative, so here I was in the psychiatric program for crazy people, a somewhat humiliating situation. You see, the alcohol recovery program carried a higher status, and a definite hierarchy existed in the hospital. Everyone knew that the chemically dependent patients were a much better class of people than the psychiatric patients. I myself remembered the condescending remarks the recovery patients made about the psychiatric patients. We all had the feeling that "at least I ain't a psych patient." I, on the other hand, had sobered up to graduate to the psych program. Life had played a cruel trick on me.

Most of the staff had changed, but a few of the same counselors and assistants were still around. Randy, a curly headed Hispanic man, who reminded me of Johann Sebastian Bach, worked primarily in the program for chemically dependent patients, but he occasionally worked with the psych patients. One day, he showed us a videotape of a Vietnam veteran who had suffered serious wounds after a phosphate grenade destroyed half his face and severely burned his fingers and arms. This heroic veteran had overcome his tragic losses and learned to play the piano. We saw the tape of him playing a phenomenal rendition of *Danny Boy*. Randy showed this videotape to encourage the psych patients to overcome their handicaps. I ended up thinking that I was sure no hero and hadn't made any great sacrifices for anyone, much less my country.

I maintained a journal to keep a record of events as they happened in order to keep a check on my memory, which had become so bad. Keeping a journal allowed me to verify that I was in touch with reality. With all of my deteriorated abilities, I had a great fear of losing my mind. At no time did any doctor sit down to tell me that this condition was not progressive; therefore, I stumbled around from day to day worried about losing myself to the sinister clutches of some complicated neurological disease.

I believed that schizophrenia was a possibility, although based on my undergraduate classes I doubted that it was the case. However, without a written record, how could I monitor my thought processes? At this point, no one on staff appeared to be monitoring me—at least I was unaware of any.

It took a significant amount of time to write neatly in my notebook each day, and I often became upset when I formed letters incorrectly or missed words in sentences. These difficulties happened frequently, and I'd end up scribbling angrily and tearing the paper. I would curse and become quite upset. My journal entries often were illegible, but sometimes when I took great pains to slowly and carefully form my letters, the writing was somewhat readable.

There was a young, Native American woman named Nora, in the psych ward who happened to have some math texts with her. I don't know why she had them, but perhaps she was studying for a high school graduate equivalency or something of that nature. At any rate, she would loan me her math texts from time to time, and I attempted to rehabilitate my ability to think by working on math problems and then check myself against the answer sheet. After years of teaching math, I'd been reduced to this!

On July 18, sometime before 7:00 AM, I carefully penciled in the following entry in my journal:

"I woke up last night with despair, but I remembered that I should live and I really want to be shelved. (*I believe that I had intended on writing don't want to be shelved, but I skipped a word again*) Greg came and saw me last night during visiting hours. That really lifted my spirits. I want to live [sic] I felt a little dull this morning. My goals (*undecipherable from this point forward*).

Later that day, when Greg came during visiting hours again, he left me a card with a Bible verse on it, Ephesians 3:20-21: *Now unto him that is able to do exceedingly abundantly above all that we ask or think, according to the power that worketh in us, unto him be glory in the church by Christ Jesus throughout all ages, world without end. Amen.* During the past years of my recovery from alcoholism, Greg was a very important spiritual advisor to me.

***

I began to wonder if God was really powerful enough to do something beyond what I was able to ask or think. Could it be possible? Was it true? It gave me something to think about.

During occupational therapy each day, I spent my time attempting to color and paint in order to focus on my fine motor skills. I tried to be bold and use bright colored markers and paint. I colored an outlined owl with brown, black, and yellow magic markers, attempting to stay within the lines—a tedious task, and one that didn't always go well. It must have been a sad picture to see a thirty-four year old graduate student attempting to do childhood coloring exercises, but I was determined to work on my fine motor skills.

One of the pictures I colored in was of a parrot, but that reminded me of my diving trip to San Carlos and of the brightly colored papier-mâché parrot I had purchased there. That plunged me into sadness, because I'd never again go to San Carlos, and scuba diving would be out of the question. I wanted to cry, but the tears would not flow from my wounded spirit. I wondered if my brain damage had something to do with my inability to cry, or perhaps it was something that could be corrected with all of the group therapy sessions.

Overall, my determination to work on my fine-motor skills was sporadic and depended on fatigue factors and wild mood swings. Still, Dr. Clairemont had not prescribed antidepressants or other psychotropic drugs, which was a relief because I was frightened about taking any type of medications.

Various counselors, including a man named Michael, who had been my ex-wife's counselor some years before, ran the group therapy sessions. I had met him before, and he seemed like a very pleasant professional. Michael led some of the groups in which I participated, and many of the patients shared their feelings and worked on personal goals, while others talked about living with some of the side effects of the psychotropic meds they were taking.

These sessions were difficult, because I became consumed with monitoring my ability to remember, and I was always saddened when I saw poor results. For example, I'd look around the circle and try to remember people's names, but I couldn't do it. For years I'd memorized the names of pupils in several classrooms, but now I couldn't remember the names of a handful of men and women in these groups.

At night and during my free time, I attempted to read stories from *Readers' Digest,* but during my stay at the hospital I only managed two short articles. Again, I noticed that I had trouble staying on the same line, and if I lost my place on the page I'd have to start over from the beginning.

Many of the group therapy sessions included wordy handouts, but even if I had wished to study the ones on chemical dependency, over-achieving children, or any of the various inspirational poems and writings, my lack of ability to focus and remember what I read prohibited gaining anything useful. The topics ranged from studies about chemical dependency to dealing with emotions and the many psychological aspects of depression and medication regulation. Again, I had lucked out, as Dr. Clairemont had not prescribed anything. I was glad that I had not started drinking during this ordeal, and I didn't believe that medication would be good for me either.

One homework assignment in group therapy was entitled *Please Hear What I Am Not Saying.* I completed the written portion with the following:

I was a man full of strength and energy, but now am a case for the books. I was lied to by so many people, that I now don't know what to believe regarding my condition. I was once a brilliant man.

I used to play the piano, guitar, and bass quite well, but now I am uncoordinated and can play very little. At 34, music, my one love of life, is gone. If I could trust that I could regain this ability, I would go for it;

however, I can't believe it.

My one cousin, an R.N., laughed at me when I suggested suicide, and she told me not to do it indoors because it would [sic] messy.

The Bluffs could be good!

Even today, it's sad to think that this simple piece of writing took me an hour to complete.

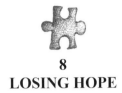

8
LOSING HOPE

During my stay at the hospital, I kept walking in an attempt to improve my gait dysfunction and my balance problems. And that's how I met Virgil, a Native American boy, most likely only thirteen or fourteen years old and dressed in typical heavy metal fashion, including blue jeans and t-shirts covered with images of death. His long black hair draped over his head, usually covering his eyes. A patient in the chemical dependency program, he never shared exactly what had landed him in the hospital. I'm certain, though, that he hadn't chosen this admittance of his own free will, and I suspected that he'd had a scrape with the law.

Virgil would occasionally join me in the gym, as I walked the perimeter for the allotted hour of recreation time. Because walking and talking were a bit too much for me, I would listen as he told me about some of his problems. I did mention that I'd quit doing any drugs many years before and that I had been free from alcohol for almost three years. He listened in disbelief when I related that I was into music, and that I was an electric bass player. I suppose I looked pretty ragged, as my hair had not been cut in many months and I still sported a curly beard.

I found comfort in listening to Virgil, and my spiritual program directed me to help those attempting to escape the clutches of addiction. As for Virgil, I truly believed he'd made a wrong turn with his life and that with the right influence he would avoid much of the heartache I and so many others had experienced. He reminded me of so many struggling students in the support groups I'd once facilitated at the junior high—that seemed like so long ago. Walking with Virgil helped me quit thinking about myself, a good thing, because I'd become exhausted with self analysis. Virgil and I were in different programs at the hospital, and years separated us in age, but I always listened if he sought me out.

Virgil also hung out with Jarrod, a seventeen-year-old, who had already been down the road just a little too far to get better through a simple recovery program. Besides, he looked rough and didn't seem to welcome help or guidance. He had the attitude of a young person who had all the answers, and they could be found in a bottle, a joint, or some other drug. In addition, Jarrod acted in hateful, mean ways with other patients. Sadly, Virgil often ran around with him because the facility didn't have many teenage patients.

A couple of days into my stay at the hospital, "Majestic Dave" showed up. He'd started drinking again and come back to the facility to sober up. He was an average chess player, but I beat him every time. Playing chess did confirm that I had abilities in long-term memory, as my previously learned chess skills were intact. As a matter of fact, I'd been the county chess champion about eight years earlier. Although I still had chess skills, playing the game drained me emotionally and mentally, and I no longer had the physical stamina to concentrate for the hours required to play in a tournament. When I played with Majestic Dave, I monitored my skills and just let him run his mouth. I managed to keep my cool, despite his arrogance.

Although I attempted to talk to people, I often fell into deep despair. I wasn't on medication yet, and nothing seemed to be helping me. One day, during group therapy we had a sentence completion assignment. We were told to say the first thing that came to mind without thinking it over. My answers certainly were revealing. Here's a sample:

I like *death*.

To me the future looks *bleak!*

I believe I have the ability to *(extremely dark and almost illegible scribbling) kill myself*.

My secret ambition in life *is to kill myself*.

Such was my state of mind. I listened to others in the group, but I could never retain anything about their problems—it was impossible to hang onto new information. Likewise, while I understood the loneliness of my self-inflicted brain injury, no one seemed to be able to understand the hell in which I functioned every day. I was unable to explain myself to anyone, and I had the feeling that no one in the hospital believed a word I was saying. To them, I was just another crazy person in the psych group. My loneliness never led to tears, because anger was the only emotion that I could feel—and I could feel it well.

Another young man, Tommy, was strapped into a wheelchair. Tommy's face was grotesquely distorted, and he had very little control of his arms and legs. An orderly had to assist him with meals. Tommy didn't talk, and he didn't seem to understand anything others said, although he made grunting sounds and frequently laughed loudly. I recognized that Tommy was truly trapped in the holding area of life, soon to be shelved in a human warehouse somewhere.

Tommy triggered overwhelming guilt in me. How could I be so self-centered as to think that my life was such a pitiful plight that I needed to be shelved? Still, no matter how I tried to encourage myself by thinking about Tommy's tragic condition, I couldn't lift myself up for long.

On one occasion, Jarrod approached Tommy and began harassing him, with Virgil following close behind and mimicking Jarrod's words and actions. The two boys circled Tommy and began chanting "Demon from hell, demon from hell," followed by attempts to imitate the distorted sounds of electric guitars and pounding rock drums. Then they began hitting Tommy's wheelchair with their fists and they kept it up until I blurted, "Cut that crap out!"

They both stopped with surprise at hearing my angry voice. Jarrod glared at me. I didn't like him, and the feeling was mutual. The hatred in his eyes and his demeanor made him look demonic, and I was especially concerned that he'd led Virgil into being cruel to another human being who could not defend himself. The entire situation disturbed me.

One evening, almost the entire ward was present in the gym, and we divided up into teams to play volleyball. I was in one of my more positive moods, and as I played I tried to compensate for my poor balance; giving it 110%, as they say. Jarrod was forced to play on the "psych" team rather than the "cds" (chemical dependency); he resented that and made no attempt to hide it.

I was not a valuable player, but I hobbled around the court and worked hard to keep my balance. But Jarrod came over to me and began ordering me around. "Move the f**ck over," he yelled.

"No!" I attempted to keep my eye on the ball, and I resented this unruly, vulgar teenager ordering me around.

"I said move the f**ck over, you f**cking psycho from hell," Jarrod yelled.

"I told you no, you f**cking bastard," I yelled back, not yielding one inch to him.

The recreation director came across the gym just in time to prevent a big fight. My anger had taken complete control of me, but I was also convinced that Jarrod was ready to kill me. Luckily, the director broke up the match and sent us all back to the ward.

I stumbled to my room that night, exhausted from the day. I curled up on the narrow mattress, and after pulling the thin white sheet and soft blanket up around my body, I fell into a deep sleep. Suddenly, I heard the sound of someone crawling on the floor of my private room. Was this a dream? I abruptly sat up in my bed. A voice whispered, but I could not discern the words. Then I saw a shadowy presence crawling on the floor next to my bed.

I heard Virgil whisper in broken "reservation" English, "You have only one bed in here." Long pause. "I can't sleep. I'm afraid. Would you come over to my room?"

Without thinking it through, I said, "Sure."

Virgil went to the doorway and said, "Shhh…I'll have to make sure no one is looking."

He quickly crossed the hall and went into the same room I'd stayed in for chemical dependency treatment in 1988. Because of that, it felt like a sacred and holy place. In that room, I had truly turned my life around when I asked God to come into my life and help me stay away from the booze. Even in my current confused state of mind, I remembered the night I had a spiritual experience, when I visualized the old drunk Dan and said goodbye to him.

Reentering that room felt like returning to my own personal holy shrine of spiritual conversion. Part of that conversion meant I was to help others, and that moment, Virgil seemed to be reaching out to me. I stood wobbling at the door awaiting the hand signal from Virgil so I could sneak across the hallway without getting caught. I began to enjoy this with a spirit of childish innocence. This was the most fun I'd had since the accident.

I finally stumbled across the hall with my blue bedspread in my hands. When I got to Virgil's room, I noticed the extra bed did not have a pillow, so I sent Virgil back across to my room to get one. Finally, each of us crawled onto our separate beds and began to whisper quietly.

"I wish you were my roommate," he said. "Could you help me do my laundry?"

"Sure," I said.

The moon was rising over the bluffs, and its beams shone brightly into the room. Virgil continued to whisper, but I became totally relaxed and began to fall asleep.

Suddenly there was a knock at the door, and Virgil whispered, "Hit the floor."

He pointed to the space between the two beds, and I moved awkwardly toward the floor.

"Is Dan in there?" an unidentified voice asked.

"Yes." I picked up my bedspread and pillow and stumbled toward the doorway. I knew we had been caught. One of my former high school students from a nearby town and two other women were at the door.

A young and pleasant staff woman firmly said, "You were assigned a room."

"Yes ma'am. I won't do it again. I'll stay in my room."

I stumbled back across the hallway to my room, where I slept until morning. However, I missed breakfast and was late for my first group therapy session. It was odd that no one had been sent to awaken me. Something was different. I could sense it in the air. I felt as if I'd become the butt of someone's joke, and everyone was treating me differently. The nagging symptoms, the dizziness, slurred speech, slow thinking, and such, seemed particularly magnified that morning.

In my mind, I questioned if what had happened in the night had really taken place. If so, I didn't seem to be in any trouble.

Mid-morning, I was ushered to a small office just off the main ward to meet with Dr. Collar, an associate of Dr. Clairemont's, who had conducted various psychological assessments with me during my stay at Sunrise. I hoped he had news about the extensive testing he'd done with me, or maybe he had some insight into my mental condition. I came to the meeting eager to hear what he had to say, but I soon found myself feeling like some junior high kid in the principal's office.

"Mr. Greathouse, you know you are not supposed to be in another patient's room," he barked.

"Yes, I do know that, and it won't happen again."

"I also heard you had a little problem on the volleyball court the other evening," he said in a scolding tone.

I drew a blank, not immediately remembering the incident with Jarrod, and confused that Dr. Collar would have even known about it. This conversation seemed to be going nowhere fast, and I was becoming more paranoid with each passing second. He then asked me what I thought about Jarrod.

Remembering how many young Native Americans wound up dying at an early age because of alcohol-related incidents, I said, "Well, you know…he won't make it."

"What exactly do you mean by that?" he asked.

"Well, you know…he'll wind up dead," I replied.

That was the end of my short visit with Dr. Collar.

Just after lunchtime, Michael, the counselor, came to the dining room and told me to come with him. I followed him through the double locked doors of the ward, where two policemen stood next to the desk.

"Mr. Greathouse, we need you to sign some papers for your release," one of the policemen said in a calm, soft voice.

"Release me?" I thought I was hearing things.

"We can't help you here," Michael said, "and we need to send you on to the state mental facilities. If you will, please just sign here." He pointed to a line on the paper.

A numb, but at the same time hot, feeling flushed all over my body. I thought I might become sick. But what choice did I have? I was in no condition to review what I was signing. I had to trust Michael. I knew him from my previous stay, and he was not a high-pressure, used car salesperson personality. Besides, something had to change; this stay at Sunrise was not working out well. I signed the papers.

As the officers pulled my arms behind my back to handcuff me, one said, "Sorry, we have to do this."

"That's all right," I said quietly.

Michael handed the officer a copy of a document and told him to give it to me at the detention center.

I sat in the back of the police car as the pleasant officer drove me away. I did not look back at the hospital. As the officer drove up through the valley toward the detention center, I listened to his country music playing on the radio. The sun was shining into the squad car, and my mind drifted to happier times when I used to play some of those very same songs in clubs and bars. I loved watching people dance, and I particularly enjoyed meeting lovely young women. Those days were gone. I was one step closer to being shelved, but literally along for the ride now. I felt no shame, and little fear. I had long since given up on my life.

At the station, the officers took me into the booking area, where they removed the handcuffs and I was fingerprinted. Several documents exchanged hands between the booking officers and the patrolman who had been my chauffeur for the past twenty minutes. Then I was taken to a cell, referred to as a mental hold cell, but it was actually a drunk tank.

I had been to this detention center once before, but only because the lead guitar player in one of my bands had worked here and had taken the whole band on a tour of the center. I remember him showing us the small drunk tanks reserved for the unruly, intoxicated detainees and directing us through the maze of hallways.

I sat down on the bed in the cell and opened the folded paper that Michael had told the officer to hand me. I began to freak out a bit as I read the following:

Certification for Emergency Mental Health Evaluation
I hereby certify that I am a physician licensed to practice in the State of New Mexico, and it is my belief that Dan Greathouse suffers from a mental disorder and as a result presents a likelihood of serious harm to himself/herself and/or others and that immediate detention is necessary to prevent such harm.

The grounds for my belief are as follows: The patient is having active thoughts of killing people. He has had ongoing homicidal and suicidal ideation since the time of admission. The patient has now identified a potential victim who is an inpatient in this same facility. The patient has violated ward limits by entering late at night the room of an underage male which constitutes infraction of ward rules and subjects the underage patient to potential risk. Overall patient's behavior is becoming more difficult to control and he is clearly verbalizing a fear that may escalate to a point where he could not control his aggressive/homicidal thoughts.

Dated 7/26/91 Signed by Physician (M.D. or D.O.) *illegible*

I sat in shock for what seemed like several hours, reading and rereading this paper, the glimmers of understanding coming through. The seed had already been planted for me to doubt my sanity, and this document was about to push me over the edge.

Ongoing homicidal thoughts? That was new. I'd not considered killing people. How in the world had this been determined? The paper said that I had "now identified a potential victim who is an inpatient." This statement was particularly disturbing, and I really began to doubt my sanity.

64

Prior to this incident, I still believed that I had decompression illness, but now I was entertaining the thought that I might indeed be a paranoid schizophrenic. My God, what do I do now that I am truly losing my mind? How would I be able to determine when I had finally crossed over into a darker place than I had ever imagined?

I did not break down and cry and wail uncontrollably. If that were to happen, they would consider it proof that I was insane, and I was unwilling to play a role in some Hollywood script about a crazy person. Perhaps, I thought, this paper was trumped-up information to ensure that I would be shelved. Hadn't Dr. Clairemont assured me that he could make that happen? I could still hear his words and see the grin on his face.

"Don't worry," he had told me, "I can get you shelved. No problem."

The part about having trouble controlling my suicidal thoughts was a given. However, if I had identified a person I was going to kill, and I had no idea who that person was, then I really was in trouble. My God! Is this what it is like to have delusions? Is this what it is like to be a paranoid schizophrenic? Sitting all alone in the cell, I was truly humbled.

9

JAIL THERAPY

Late July heat blanketed the inmates in the stuffy cells. The grimy concrete floor contrasted with the puke-yellow blocks that constituted the lower half of the six-by-ten-foot drunk tank. A great poet may have provided a glamorous image of people leaving footprints in the sand after they depart from this life, but the sights and smells of that cell were a far cry from a peaceful shore on some lovely ocean beach. But hey, what could I expect? After all, this was a drunk tank for unreasonable, violent, and intoxicated individuals who needed to be removed from the social stream. It doubled as a solitary confinement mental hold cell, including its own tiny window with a hinged shutter from which a jailor could periodically check to make certain that the detainee had not stuck his head in the metal toilet in an attempt to commit suicide by drowning. Actually, if anyone were to die in this cell it was going to be from heat exhaustion or the food.

One dusty vent mockingly pointed down into the cell from its perch near the top of the plastered section of the wall, taunting me with the empty hope of cool air. Instead, the lukewarm flow was only noticeable because of the strings of dark green dust tentacles that waved back and forth from time to time. A single military-issue wool blanket lay tossed in a heap at one end of a stainless steel ledge attached to the wall. It appeared more like an autopsy table than a place for sleeping. The ledge, or shelf, connected to the wall. It was barely wide enough for one sleeping human. No soap was near the basin or anywhere in the Spartan six-by-ten foot cell, but thank God there was a roll of toilet paper.

Fluorescent lights glared down into the cell from the ceiling. One wired-over glass window, about four-by-eight inches in size occasionally allowed some natural light into the cell when the doors to the booking and fingerprinting area were open to process more inmates into the detention center. Sadly, business in the processing area was particularly heavy in this jurisdiction. In fact, the county held the record for the highest per capita number of drunk-driving related fatalities in the state of New Mexico.

The nearby reservation, which restricted the legal sale of alcoholic beverages, accounted for some of the DUIs, but the local politicians and newspapers downplayed the number of non-reservation inhabitants who contributed to the out-of-control epidemic. In reality, this was not only a

"Native American" problem, but crossed all racial lines in the county.

Since I couldn't see a clock, I approximated time by noting when the lukewarm coffee and powdered eggs arrived for breakfast, and two bologna sandwiches with a cup of sugary red Kool-Aid indicated noon. Somewhat tastier fare signaled dinnertime and the approach of evening. I wasn't allowed outside for a walk or to see other inmates or attend a church service, so I was truly alone.

At first, I was relieved to be away from the mental hospital; far from the Sunrise psychiatrist, Dr. Clairemont. Although he had not yet prescribed anything for me, I feared eventually being turned into a zombie with psychotropic meds. I'd become disillusioned with him, and apparently, after spending a few minutes with me, he thought the state mental hospital was the best place. Although I had arrived at the hospital with the intent of becoming warehoused, I really wanted help. I was deeply disappointed that he had not personally tried to help me. He had met with me during the initial intake, briefly saw me in passing one day, and performed a completely irrelevant and rather embarrassing hernia examination on another day. Sometimes I felt relieved to be out of his evil clutches and at other times I thought he sold me down the river. His words on the paper that justified my removal from the hospital would haunt me for years to come.

Quickly, my new location unveiled itself as the living nightmare it was intended to be. It did not take me long to figure out that I was in a bad place, especially after I endured four hot July days without a shower, wearing the same smelly orange jail overalls. Each day slowly oozed down the dark drain that sat in the middle of my cell. I waited for visiting day and the court hearing to determine my move to the state mental hospital. Somehow I knew that the medical treatment of my condition would only become more barbaric as I was traded from a private institution to the poorly run state facilities, but I was mostly too numb to care anymore. Still, I paced back and forth in the cell for hours, limping in my now-famous off balance shuffle, muttering under my breath, "Please help me, God." I also used my one allowed collect phone call each day to talk to my parents.

The first phone call came as a shock to my father, as I told him what happened to land me in jail. When Dad asked me for more information, I explained that I had not done anything wrong, but I could still sense the anxiety on the other end of the line four hundred miles away. The one and only time I had called my father from jail was on a false arrest for stealing gasoline when I was a rowdy college student. I'd never been arrested for drunk driving during my horrible drinking career.

Naturally, my father was upset and asked several times if I had hit or injured anyone. I admitted that I had violated the ward rules, but I could not believe that such an action would have required handcuffs and a jail cell as a consequence.

"Just stay calm," my dad said. "Your mother and I are going to see what we can do." I later learned that my father called the hospital to get more information.

So many times I have taken my supportive family for granted. Even with all our faults, my family has always been there for me through thick and thin. During the darkest hours, my parents prayed for me and they were actively involved in helping out. Where would my life have ended up without their love and devotion?

This crucial turning point in my life would lead me to a deeper understanding of God and His love for us all. I recalled the story of Jesus leaving the flock to rescue the one lost lamb. I was a bewildered and lost lamb at this point in my life. Dad's voice was reassuring, and I hung on to an ever so slight belief that somehow he and Mom would come up with some way to help me through this ordeal.

Although I was an adult and they were not legally responsible for me, my folks still were upset that they had not been contacted. In retrospect, I hope that these laws and procedures are changed one day so that next of kin could be notified in cases like mine. When my dad finally spoke to the administrator of Sunrise, Douglas King, he was told of the certification for emergency mental health evaluation, which would be used in my court hearing. My father asked if I had molested or injured any patient in the facility. Mr. King's answer was an unequivocal no.

My father focused on certain words in the certification of emergency mental health evaluation: *potential risk, homicidal, suicidal, violated, and infraction.* The idea that they'd put me in jail infuriated my father. Wasn't Sunrise supposed to help patients with problems like mine? My father asked if one of the doctors or counselors would see me during my next seven days in solitary confinement. He let Mr. King know that I should be receiving some type of support from their trained workers and not just the basic services of jail employees. But Sunrise did not make any effort to attend to me during my incarceration, and my father has always believed this to be negligence on their part.

After one day, I had trouble accepting my solitary confinement, and then I learned that my court hearing was a week away. During a phone call, Dad explained this to me as best he could, and he assured me that he and Mom were coming up to see me in the jail. This one fact gave me hope.

At one point, I asked the guard if it was possible to post bond and get out of this place. I had money, and even if I hadn't, I believed that my parents would have posted bond money for my release. But then I'd remember that I didn't have anywhere to go, and I could barely drive my truck for any significant distance. Besides, I continued to feel awful, with no improvement of my symptoms. At any rate, I soon learned that no one could post bond money for mental hold patients.

While dialing my father's phone number, I'd noticed a pencil sketch of a wanted man taped to the glass window of the control room. It was quite haunting and like looking at a picture of myself. This felt terrible, since the man in the sketch was wanted for a series of rapes that had occurred north of the city. But I couldn't get over the fact that the sketched person looked like me—except for the eye color. I began to worry even more about what was going on here in the detention center. Furthermore, it had been almost a week and I was still in the mental hold cell. Something was not right, but I just could not put my finger on it.

"You have to hang in there, Dan," my father calmly talked with me.

"What else can I do?" I stammered a reply.

"We're coming up tomorrow to see you," he continued.

Although I had neither a clock nor a calendar to help me out, I struggled each day to maintain a concept of time, so I could prepare for my court hearing on Thursday. I counted blocks on the wall to help me keep a mental calendar. Unfortunately, I had no idea about the nature of the court hearing, although I figured I would need to defend myself against the allegations of homicidal ideations—and find out exactly who the potential victim might have been.

Naturally, I was concerned about memory problems appearing on the witness stand, and nagging thoughts about possible schizophrenia continued to wear on my nerves. Another haunting thought occurred to me. What if they thought I was the suspected rapist? How would I defend myself against such absurd allegations?

Later that afternoon, the guards came by and pulled me out of my cell to be photographed. I stood against a wall near the booking area, looking pretty rough with my beard and unkempt hair. Hell, I had not had a shower in almost a week now. The photographer had me face forward, then turn to one side, and then the other way. It was not the typical jail photography session where the inmate holds up the numbers.

About a week into my incarceration, a young guard walked by my cell and looked in the window. Then a familiar voice asked, "Mr. G. is that you?"

"Yes, and who are you?"

"It's me, Richard."

I strained to look out the window and saw the friendly face of Richard Brewer, one of my former math students at the nearby high school where I had taught five years before. "Richard Brewer! What have you been up to?" I attempted to carry on a conversation as if we were two people casually reunited by chance in some local restaurant.

"Mr. G., is there anything I can get for you?" Richard asked.

This was so different from what I'd become used to in the jail that I even wondered if Richard was a figment of my imagination. His voice resounded with the same respect he'd shown me as his teacher. In fact, most of my students had referred to me as Mr. G. instead of Mr. Greathouse.

"Could I have a shower, Richard? I have gone for several days without one."

"Sure, Mr. G. Let me get everything ready, and I'll be back to get you."

I waited, almost certain that his supervisors would fill him in on my status. But, much to my surprise and joy, Richard came for me. My heart raced at the thought of a shower with soap and a change of clothes.

Richard rattled the key into the metal lock, swung open the squeaky metal door, and said, "Step out in front of me, Mr. G., and I'll tell you which way to go."

The next few minutes passed like a nightmare, echoing with the sound of footsteps walking through a maze of corridors and passageways, like Theseus must have encountered when he fought the Minotaur. It seemed that my entire existence was reduced to warm water and a white bar of soap. I had arrived at the gates of heaven. If only the water would cleanse my damaged brain—I would have been so much more relieved.

I scrubbed myself from head to toe, diligently attempting to hold on to the bar of soap, only dropping it a few dozen times! How had I ever taken showers for granted? As I dried myself, I was amazed at how soft the clean white towel felt. Too bad my blanket back in the cell didn't feel like this.

Around that time, another one of my former high school students, now a guard, helped me out by giving me a small notepad and pencil. I'd never been happier that I'd gotten along well with almost all of the students I had ever taught. I used the notebook to make notes for my court hearing, and the writing itself seemed to help me—it felt like a reality check. I wrote the history of what happened to me and also copied some verses from a Bible I'd managed to get my hands on at the detention center.

One day when I could not reach my parents by phone, I called my high school friend, Lee Ann. She was surprised to hear from me, and shocked when I told her what was going on and began praying for me over the phone, offering again some small measure of hope that I'd be cured. Although I didn't share her optimism, I was still glad to know that someone with such faith was praying for me.

On the day before my hearing, I was moved to a new cell. I was ready for that, and for another change of clothes. The orange jumpsuit was pretty disgusting by now, and the July heat did not help matters. My new cell was much smaller, but I still paced back and forth, because I continued to hope that if I practiced my walking enough, I would regain my balance. I also paced to relieve stress while I said the simple prayer over and over, "Please help me, God."

One morning, I heard friendly voices outside my cell. I could hear a man and a woman talking and laughing.

"Hello," I stammered.

"Hello, Mr. Greathouse," the female voice said.

I asked what time it was, and was told it was about three.

"In the afternoon?" I asked, wondering to myself how I had slept such a long time.

"No, three o'clock in the morning," the woman said with a laugh.

Despite the time, we continued to talk back and forth, and the two guards introduced themselves as Lloyd and Martha. They were a husband-wife team who had been working at the detention center for several years. Apparently, they had been on vacation, but once back, they changed things for me somewhat because they were very nice. Lloyd took me to the detention center library to check out some books. Wow! I could look at all the books on the shelves without interruption. After being locked down for so many days, I suddenly found myself in heaven again. First, the shower and now this library tour! Lloyd acted as though he had all the time in the world.

As Lloyd and Martha continued to talk with me, I eventually asked for the date. I learned that it was August 1st, a date with great importance to me—my third year anniversary of sobriety. Two and a half months had passed since my brain injury at Lake Powell. I ended up telling the couple about my scuba diving accident and all that had happened, although I didn't supply many details about my stay at Sunrise. Lloyd and Martha appeared to genuinely care and said they would pray for me.

My parents drove the eight or so hours to be with me for my court hearing. Realistically, I didn't see what they could do to help, especially since it looked as if I'd be institutionalized. I knew that would break their hearts. Still, anticipating their visit gave me something to look forward to, and this filled my heart with childlike hope. I ate breakfast that morning with my spirits high. Suddenly, I heard someone at my cell door and I felt excited. Visitation time had finally arrived.

"Mr. Greathouse, will you please come with me?" the jailer said, as his brass-colored key rattled in the keyhole of the cold, tan metal door. The long bolt slid open and came to a final thud; the sound as disturbing as fingernails scraping on a blackboard.

I followed the jailor down the hallway into the maze of the detention center. We rounded the corner, and he led me into a room with two men—very odd.

"Mr. Greathouse, please take a seat," the "official" man asked.

I sat down at the table in a room that didn't look at all like a visitation room. My heart sank. Had my parents been in an accident?

"Mr. Greathouse, my name is Detective Radnor and this is Captain Robert Layton," he said, pointing to the other man. "We are here to ask you some questions about a woman who was murdered in your neighborhood."

As Detective Radnor continued talking, my mind, already numb, became even more so, and the feeling spread through my entire body. First, the composite sketch of a suspected rapist who looked uncomfortably similar to me, then the photography session with the detention center photo team, and now this!

"Where were you on July 10?" the detective asked.

"I am not sure right now, but I think I was with my folks," I replied.

"We are aware that you're in trouble, and maybe we can be of help," he said.

It quickly dawned on me that they had no help to offer, but were gathering information so they could try to pin a murder on me.

"We have sources that tell us your mother is the type of woman who would lie for her sons to get them out of trouble," Detective Radnor said.

The comment shocked me. Now I was a murder suspect. Was I more seriously mentally ill than I ever imagined?

"Take a look at these pictures," the detective barked. "She was a professional race walker." He showed me pictures of bloodstained walking shorts and a colorful sports top drenched in blood. I don't recall him showing me a picture of the actual victim, but at this point I was doing rather well just to maintain my balance in the chair and avoid passing out from shock. I sat in silence.

"She was murdered on July 10, early in the morning," he continued. "She was murdered two blocks over from your home on Camina Placer. Have you ever seen a woman competitive walker in your neighborhood?"

I did not have the mental capacity to carry on a logical argument against this intelligent and persistent detective. I couldn't remember where I was on July 10, but I did not remember murdering anyone! If I had been able to think clearly, I could have explained how ridiculous it was for the police even to be considering me as a suspect. How could a person in my condition, unable to maintain his balance, much less overcome his ataxia and gate dysfunction, catch up to and overcome a professional race walker?

"Besides, someone called in to tell us that you are an extremely violent man," he continued.

Completely overwhelmed, all I could do was sit there, looking at the pictures of the bloodstained clothing and shake my head in disbelief.

"Is there something you wish to tell us, Mr. Greathouse?" asked Captain Layton.

"I remember seeing a woman walker, but that was quite some time back," I stammered. Had I actually remembered seeing such a person, or were these men planting a memory in my damaged brain?

"You don't have anything to hide do you?" Radnor asked.

"No."

"Well, then, could we search your house and vehicle?" Layton asked.

"Sure," I replied, hoping and praying to God that I had not really done something that I could not remember, and that they wouldn't find something to further implicate me with this hideous accusation.

"You know, if you could help us out here, we might be able to help you out. Things could go a little better for you if you confess the truth. We know about your court hearing this afternoon," Radnor added.

"Can you think of anything you might like to confess?" Layton asked.

"I can't think of anything," I muttered. Why did everyone else know more about what was going on than I did?

"Well, here's my card in case you think of anything. Just call me." Radnor handed me his official city police card with address and phone number. Then he told the guard to take me back to my cell.

I had a whole new set of things to worry about. On top of all my problems, the court hearing was this afternoon and I wasn't ready. I furiously scratched notes on the back of Radnor's card and then on the yellow pad. I penciled in names and dates as best I could, guessing at the days and times of everything I'd done for two months. It came out a jumbled, incoherent mess. I could provide no proof of my whereabouts on July 10.

Finally, it was time for my visit, which took place in a room with a long, double-paned glass with telephones positioned along the way, enough for eight inmates to visit at the same time. Expecting to see my parents, I was pleasantly surprised to see my good friend, Rick Hedges. There he stood, big and tall, in his Texas cowboy boots and cowboy hat. He smiled and laughed, bringing bright sunshine into my day that had turned to crap. We both reached for the phones.

"How's it going, DG?" he asked.

"Well, I'm hanging in there, Rick."

Rick said that he had friends in the jail, and he'd told them to take good care of me. He also said that he couldn't be at my court hearing, but he reassured me that everything would be okay.

"I need all the help I can get," I said.

Rick left because my parents were waiting, and he didn't want to take up their time. He smiled, and I am sure that if I did not smile outwardly, I was smiling inwardly to myself to have such a good friend.

Finally, my parents arrived at the glass barrier. With tears in my eyes, I said, "At least I'm three years sober today."

"Oh, that's right," my mother said, her face reflecting her understanding of the importance of the day.

From then on, I lost it as I frantically explained that I needed help remembering where I was on July 10, because the police were trying to frame me for murder.

"You were at home with us," my dad said in a reassuring tone.

"Can you prove it?" I asked as if pleading for my life—and I was most assuredly doing just that.

"The court hearing this afternoon will not be about that," my mother said. My father added that they'd been working with an assistant district attorney to get me out of the state facilities and into Urban Memorial Psychiatric Hospital about four hours away.

As if not hearing (and the connection was very bad), I pleaded with them to help me, protesting yet again that I hadn't murdered anyone.

"Of course you didn't. You were with us," Mom said.

"Time's up!" one of the guards barked.

"Just stay in the boat, son," Dad said.

Much later, I learned that my parents couldn't understand me on the bad phone system. They actually had no idea what was going on with the murder investigation in which I was supposedly a primary suspect. They didn't realize that I'd been interrogated or had my picture taken in jail. After visiting my house in town later that evening, my parents found out that I'd signed a document giving the police permission to search my home. Lawrence, my acquaintance who had done some carpentry work for me, was staying in my house at the time, keeping an eye on things.

Detective Radnor had presented Lawrence with a search warrant and went through everything at my home, taking away a claw hammer and a wrench that belonged to me. They opened my mail, including my bank statements and phone bills, looking for clues. The police also confiscated a pair of Lawrence's shoes, which happened to be stained with some finish from one of his woodworking projects. The stains were mysteriously the color of blood. I'm sure the police thought they were well on the way to solving the murder.

My parents were doing quite a bit of legwork to make arrangements for my transfer to a private care facility. Their schedule included a visit with the director of Sunrise and with Dr. Clairemont. They also talked with the detectives who were working on the murder case. Dr. Clairemont and the director indicated that I had become difficult to deal with and had violated ward rules. At no time, even after being directly asked by my father, did they say that I had molested or hit anyone.

With their work completed at Sunrise, my parents proceeded with the documentation they needed to appoint themselves as my lawful attorney with full and complete power to act on my behalf. They also had to arrange for a stay in another mental health facility. I shall never be able to thank my parents enough for what they did for me during that time. They are my heroes.

My father's conversations with the police department included questions about my activities during June and early July, but my father insisted on knowing why I was even considered a suspect at all. It turned out that an anonymous phone call from a woman implicated me. Dad pressed the issue and asked Detective Radnor if such a call warranted that I be interrogated in the detention center given my mental condition—and he was upset about the search of my house and vehicle. The Farmington City police had already phoned the police department in my parents' hometown not long after the murder occurred two blocks away from my home. Radnor and my father reviewed the mileage to determine if I had, indeed, driven four hundred miles across the state, committed the murder early one morning, and then driven back across the state four hundred miles! And somehow, even with all the medical documentation regarding my current condition, the police hadn't seen clearly that I had deficits that would have made it impossible for me to commit that kind of crime. I couldn't have driven eight hundred miles round trip and committed a murder if my life depended upon it. Dad has always questioned the Farmington police policy that would allow the interrogation of a brain-damaged, suicidal person.

In the midst of all the legwork, my parents also continued meeting with the assistant district attorney, Reynaldo Montoya, who proposed an alternate plan for continued psychiatric care, avoiding the state mental hospital. My court hearing was scheduled, where crucial decisions would be made, not only affecting my life, but ultimately the course of HBOT history.

Given what happened to me over a period of years, I understand, probably better than many, how vulnerable we can all become when we suffer from an illness or injury that affects mental functioning. In my case, being "different" even led to the accusation that I committed a heinous crime. Fortunately, my parents' anxiety was put to rest when the assistant district attorney, Reynaldo Montoya, told them that I'd been cleared as a suspect in the race walker's murder. Unfortunately, they were unable to immediately communicate this to me, so I had to live with that particular mental torture a while longer. In fact, I continued to recreate a calendar from my limited memory and short-circuited thoughts.

10
MENTALLY RE-"WARDED" – AT THE SECOND PSYCH HOSPITAL

The terrible afternoon of the detention center hearing dragged on, leaving me to wait alone with only my imagination as company. Of course, I was confused and sat struggling with reconstructing the daily calendar of the summer.

Finally, I was taken to the courthouse, and although I was in handcuffs, the walk was just as glorious as I had imagined it. The sun shone down brightly on the concrete sidewalks, and the slight breeze ruffled the glimmering green cottonwood trees that towered above the facility. Thank you, God, for this! I muttered under my breath. With the sun shining on me, I was relieved to be free, even if only for the moment, from my solitary confinement cell. This was a day of reprieve, and I savored every second of my short walk from the detention center to the courtroom.

Once inside the courthouse, however, fear and hopelessness flooded into my soul, much like the feelings I had as a child when I approached the open casket of a loved one. I also felt overwhelmed by fear of the unknown, having no idea what would transpire at my hearing, or how I would defend myself. As I walked through the glass and metal doorways of the County Detention Court Center, I strained to remain focused on the beautiful outside world, even thinking that I could almost hear the Animas River flowing somewhere to the south. Not so long before, I'd been free to raft the river, rappel from the sandstone cliffs, mountain bike the canyons, and otherwise move about in God's glorious world.

Finally, we arrived at the huge double doors of the courtroom. As I looked around the room I spotted my friend Timothy, my junior high school principal, Larry Fenton, another teacher, Don Newton, who taught at the junior high, and some other relatives in addition to my parents. With my hands released from the handcuffs, I was free to wave at those who had come to support me. They waved and smiled back.

The judge was late and apologized, but I didn't mind. The delay had given me more freedom from the drab holding cell. My drifting attention suddenly came back into focus when Judge Westside addressed me. What followed was a brief exchange in which it became clear that his daughter had been a student of mine, and I joked about hoping she'd received an A in my class. The judge joked back that his daughter rarely got anything less. I thought—and hoped—I had it right, and he was the same judge who used to sport his oversized bowties when he visited the schools for conferences.

Then the light moment passed and the hearing proceeded. At the last minute, my parents had found an attorney, Suzie Hardin, to represent me. As the judge spoke, I drifted in and out of awareness. It was so difficult for me to grasp all that transpired. I did manage to follow the fact that my request involved permission to enter the alternative psychiatric facility that my parents had found. I realized that no matter where I went, I would not be the same, and that no one could help me with my damaged brain. However, it would sure be nice to end up in a place where I might be able to take a shower more than once every seven days.

"The respondent must fully realize that such an alternative placement would have to be continued for a full thirty days," the judge said, "and that he could not simply walk off the facility."

I understood all too well that I couldn't "simply" walk away from all my problems. The court proceedings continued with legal terms tossed back and forth between my attorney, the judge, and the assistant district attorney. Ms. Hardin spoke for me and I sat silent, hoping only to avoid doing anything to jeopardize my situation.

Judge Westside approved the request to send me to the new facility and wished me luck. And that was that. I certainly knew I needed more than luck. I needed a miracle.

I was allowed a few minutes to speak with Timothy and my parents and my colleagues who had come to support me. The principal and the teacher told me they hoped I'd be well in time to get back to school at the start of the next term. It was hard to say hurried goodbyes to Mom and Dad, but the guard insisted I had to go back to the small cell for the time being.

"This was the best we could do," my dad said.

Then my mother remembered to tell me I was no longer a suspect in the race walker's murder. What a relief. I'd lived in solitude with that hanging over my head for several torturous hours; more than anyone in my mental condition should have endured.

I entered the locked cell in the detention center once again, but the next morning I was scheduled to leave the jail for Urban Memorial Psychiatric Hospital. Although I had no idea what to expect, I clung to the hope of different food and a chance for regular showers. That night, the prospect of at last escaping from the jail kept me awake. I spent most of the night reading my Bible, looking over my notes, and pacing the floor asking God to help me.

The next morning, after the cold coffee and breakfast, I was handcuffed and led outside to a white van, where several other orange-uniformed detainees were lining up for a long trip south. I listened to them talk about going to the state work farm. Then, an older gentleman in cowboy boots and a light-colored cowboy hat sauntered over to the van. I thought he looked like a character in a movie with a name like Billy Joe or Joe Bob. In any case, I was the last to be motioned to the van and he directed me to sit behind him.

As we pulled out of town, across the river, and out of the canyon, the sun rose to begin its scorching of the ancient land. Shadows from the various buttes, sandstone spires, and rock formations stretched for miles across the desert. It was almost cool that morning. Then I remembered that it was August, and the previous day had been my three-year anniversary of sobriety. When I'd first become sober, I never imagined that I'd spend a sobriety anniversary in jail.

Even though I was exhausted and wanted to sleep in the van, the loud country music "Billy Joe" had blaring out of the scratchy speakers made any rest impossible. I couldn't complain, though. The driver treated me well, even attempting conversation. I suppose he wasn't afraid of me, and of course, I was harmless enough. He dropped the other inmates at the state work farm and then went on to the hospital. Once the others were gone and the van was empty, he released my hands from the cuffs.

"There, now I trust you not to do anything crazy," he said.

"I won't," I replied.

I don't remember any of the details of our conversation, but I remember it as pleasant. Finally, we left the interstate and soon pulled into the circular drive of a four-storied building.

"Well, I hope I got you here in time for lunch," he said.

I looked up at the large gray building with windows and black bars and a red tiled roof—adding at least some color to the exterior. The elm trees surrounding the building towered almost to the height of the roof itself, and the green lawn was obviously the product of dedicated groundskeepers.

The driver led me inside to a foyer that seemed more like a hotel registration area. He talked to the woman at the admissions desk. Before he left, he wished me luck. It seemed that everyone wished me luck—I guess I was the luckiest man in the world.

I signed some papers and was taken up to the fourth floor of the psychiatric hospital. The attendant was pleasant enough, and it was a relief not to see uniformed guards, but I wasn't surprised when the doors locked behind me. I knew I'd be in the lockdown area of the psych hospital. My room was such a contrast from the cell. Wow! A large bed had fluffy pillows, and outside the window were the green leaves of a huge elm tree. Even through the bars on the window, the view was magnificent. Standing in that room, I experienced something I hadn't felt in a long time. I think it was joy. I asked if I could shower, and the nurse said yes. No surprise there—I probably smelled awful. I also saw a change of clothes in my room. I later learned that my parents had brought them from Sunrise, where the staff had neatly packed my few T-shirts, Levis, socks, underwear, toiletries, and even my notebook. At last I shed the filthy, orange prison suit that had clung to my body for too many days. It was a special baptism of warm water, soap, and even shampoo. I had not washed my hair with shampoo for quite some time.

How joyous it felt to stand in the never-ending stream of shower water—even my soul felt cleansed. I hadn't felt such joy or peace in a long time. How could a simple shower bring about such an emotional response? I would have cried, but I was afraid that I might lose control and alarm the staff. Still, a few tears of joy found their way to the corners of my eyelids and fell, mixing with the warm shower water that flowed toward the drain.

After the shower, I looked into the mirror, only to be shocked by the wild-looking man staring back at me. Although clean, I had a wild look in my eyes, which brought home the reality of being in a locked ward.

When I hobbled from the shower room out into the ward, I looked around to see who might be there. One older gentleman wearing very thick glasses mumbled softly while he walked near the nurses' station and steadied himself by leaning on the countertops and tables. Other people sat around watching television or playing cards or working on jigsaw puzzles.

Two nurses sat behind the counter at the nurses' station, and a couple of psychiatric ward technicians walked about, one of whom approached me and introduced me to the gentleman with the thick glasses. I never retained their names. I was just too exhausted to learn new information. Cognitive tasks had become too demanding, and I always seemed to do worse at the end of the day, which is a classic symptom for people with brain injuries. As the day wears on, end-of-the-day fatigue brings the deficits out. I was at my best, such as it was, in the morning.

Later, alone in my room, I felt as if I'd been resurrected to a newer, albeit imperfect world. Down deep inside, I still knew I was brain-damaged, but for that moment, I felt whole and complete, warm and safe—and quite sleepy.

When I woke up the world was dark outside my window. Confused, I left the room and saw that the area was dark, with the exception of the dimly lit nurses' station to my left. I sat down in a chair and began to watch whatever program was on the television and felt wide awake. But I was soon ushered back to my room and told that since it was nighttime I was supposed to sleep. Then a nurse brought me medication in a plastic cup.

The nurse, whose manner was condescending and cold, tried to dodge answering the question, but I pressed until I learned it was Thorazine. This frightened me. My new found world of showers, clean clothes, and a nice bed had its downside, and this nurse was the face of that downside. I had no choice in this matter of medications, and I knew it. My spirits sank.

I dreaded taking the Thorazine. During my spiritual walk and recovery from alcohol, I met a man who had been to several psychiatric hospitals. He had mentioned Thorazine and talked about the "Thorazine shuffle." I had trouble enough with gait and balance, so I feared anything that would make it worse.

I ended up taking the medication, because I felt powerless not to. I remember very little else about that night, but I will never forget that nurse and her demands. Was it just because I had awakened and gone out into the dayroom to watch television? The next morning, I was in a daze. I'd never had a hangover so bad. Even my vision was blurry. The Thorazine had turned the hospital into a nightmare and left me wondering how I'd survive. I was savvy enough to understand that the nightshift motto was "drug them and put them to bed." I made up my mind never to leave my room at night. Plus, I'd learn the rules of this lock-down unit and always comply. Jail cells and Thorazine loomed as the consequences of "bad behavior."

I stumbled out into the dayroom area, where everyone gathered for breakfast. A couple of kitchen staff arrived with the metallic enclosed food cart and began setting food trays with each of the patients. Not knowing anyone, I sat alone and awaited my tray. Ah yes, I did know the elderly man who mumbled. He sat quietly by himself sipping coffee. Did I look as bad as he did? Poor old man, I thought. He probably suffered a stroke or something.

As bad as I felt, I probably would have stayed in that easy chair all day long had it not been for my appointment with the head psychiatrist, Dr. Butz. A nurse escorted me down the hallway and around the corner into a small room where a gray-haired man with an equally gray beard rose from his chair on his side of the desk. He held out his hand and introduced himself.

I did the same, although my words were quite slurred because of the Thorazine. Dr. Butz interviewed me, and once again, I ended up telling the whole story, from the scuba diving accident forward. In a stern tone, Dr. Butz explained the lockdown ward policies, and I eagerly agreed to comply with all the facility rules, knowing I'd do anything within my power to avoid being placed in a jail cell again. That was one experience I did not care to repeat, no matter what was asked of me.

Later, after another glorious shower, one of the activities directors sat with another patient and me at a round wooden table. Although I had a difficult time balancing on the chair, I attempted to participate in some sort of modified dominoes game. The shapes were hexagonal with two numbers on each side. Although the pleasant activities director explained the game to me several times, and the rules seemed basic enough, I could not seem to catch on. In the past, I had aspired to play chess professionally. Now, I sat resigned at the table, completely overwhelmed by a simple game. I could only go through the motions, too drugged and too tired to get up from the table and leave. Even in my drugged, mentally dull state, when lunchtime came, I knew the food tasted great.

Later, I met Dr. Nettleton, one of the staff psychologists. For an hour or so, Dr. Nettleton sat and talked in a corner of the dayroom. Once again, I attempted to recount my journey to this lock-down unit. He appeared to be very knowledgeable and kind, and when he noticed that I had a difficult time staying balanced on the couch, he asked if I was okay.

"Not really," I replied.

"Do you wish to tell me your feelings about what is going on?" he asked.

"They gave me Thorazine last night," I said, although I really had no feelings because I was overmedicated.

Dr. Nettleton continued to talk with me for a little bit longer, but soon he dismissed me to join the other patients in the ward. I noticed the mumbling man touching the wooden countertop at the nurses' station. He ran his hands over the dark, smooth surface, pausing near a light area of the wood.

"That's the way the brain works," an orderly standing nearby said. "You see, when the brain loses certain functions, other senses gain in strength. See how Mr. Cox holds his hands there in the lighted area? It is warmer in that area for sure. What the rest of us take for granted, Mr. Cox is now able to sense with his touch."

"Oh, I see," I said. The comments seemed odd to me, but listening to the orderly was the only thing going on. I certainly didn't want to sleep in my room, only to wake up in the middle of the night. Eventually, Mr. Cox and the orderly left the nurses' station and I ran my hands over the smooth texture and paused in the lighted area. Sure enough, the orderly was correct. I could actually feel the difference between the warm and cool portions of the countertop.

The next morning I felt a bit less fuzzy, but it was another two days before the effects of the Thorazine wore off. When I met with Dr. Nettleton again, he agreed that something had happened to me at Lake Powell, and he was happy to see that I had come out of my stupor. In fact, he said he'd been quite alarmed at my state when he first met with me.

Behind the scenes and unbeknownst to me, my parents continued to look for additional help, a pursuit that led them back to Dr. Paul Harch in New Orleans. Dad also had continued his search for delayed hyperbaric oxygen treatments for decompression illness. He'd adopted the attitude that if our modern technology had the power to put a man on the moon, then surely he could find something to help his son—and Mom agreed. It was my good luck that my parents weren't ready to give up on me, even after all that had transpired. Only three people still believed that I might have decompression illness, and the rest of the world, including the legal system, had long since written me off as just another person with some type of mental disorder.

A day later, I was told to gather things from my room because Dr. Butz and Dr. Nettleton believed I was ready for the less restricted area of the hospital. Now that was sweet music to my ears. I noted immediately that the new ward had bright colors and more windows—and more people. I felt as if I'd moved up in the world, even though I continued to be haunted by my imbalance, slurred speech, memory problems, and other neurological manifestations. Also, my moods would swing incredibly. On the one hand, I was so happy about taking hot showers and having clean clothes and good food, but then I'd experience the depression related to my brain damage.

We had more activity in this section of the psychiatric hospital, so I didn't have much unsupervised time. I attended group therapy sessions, individual counseling with Dr. Nettleton, music therapy, walking activities, and several occupational therapy groups. In addition, I was given reading materials, including a meditation book for recovering alcoholics and a twelve-step spiritual journey guide.

During that time, I longed to think or talk my way out of my problems and walk my way back into balance. Each day, no matter how pleasant my surroundings, I awakened to a world of continued nagging neurological deficits. In those moments I was convinced that I'd never get better. Although I had some bright spots during my days in this ward, for the most part I could never rise above my condition.

One day, Laura, the music therapist, asked me to play a children's melody on a small electronic keyboard. I tried my best to sight read the music, but my rhythm was completely off. I could no longer hear the music or feel the beat in my mind. I felt like poor old Mr. Cox in the lockdown ward, blindly feeling my way around the keyboard, attempting to play what I used to play with great ease. Laura told Dr. Nettleton that I had done rather well, but how could she really know? She didn't know how I had played in the past. Not knowing that I'd been a musician, she had no baseline from which to gauge my musical abilities.

My sessions with Dr. Nettleton continued, but there was never another mention of the scuba diving accident. He continued to be pleasant and encouraged me to talk openly with him. I would have talked nonstop for the next year if I thought my mental abilities would come back. According to him, I had been living my life at too fast a pace and trying to do too much: teaching during the day at the junior high school, being the onsite coordinator of the night school, playing music on the weekends, taking graduate school classes, and taking scuba diving lessons. I sensed that he believed I had experienced some type of mental breakdown brought on by the stress in my life. While I didn't believe I'd suffered a breakdown, I had the distinct feeling that what had happened to me was no accident. It was as if God interrupted my busy life and pushed His finger into my skull in order to get my attention. My recovery from alcohol had started that way, and now the scuba diving accident was a similar situation. God had my attention, but I did not know what He wanted. I had sobered up, and yet I felt as if I'd returned to the same hopeless state I had experienced when drinking. Since this felt like a cruel twist of fate, I wondered how any of this could possibly work out for the best.

Recreational activities included daily walks, which I really enjoyed. On one of the walks, I met a woman, Marcia, who was also in my group therapy sessions. Marcia, who had been admitted to the hospital in order to deal with depression, was married to a man with bipolar disorder. She told me about his extreme behavior, even once leaving her alone on the road somewhere between Tucumcari and Santa Rosa, New Mexico, just because they had an argument in the car. She tried to deal with the realities of living with him, but she often cried when she talked about him.

I shared my thoughts about obtaining a gun and killing myself, even describing how neat I'd try to be. Because Marcia was a nurse, she warned me of the horrible things that could happen if I botched the job. She'd seen patients who ended up in persistent vegetative states, hooked up to respirators and all kinds of tubing and attachments. She begged me not to even think such suicidal thoughts.

Recreation also included bocce ball. Luckily, I had learned to play this poor man's golf game at the previous mental hospital. The brightly colored balls on the green grass under the canopy of huge trees that sheltered the hospital brought a sense of happiness to my soul—or at least a sense of relief. One day, while playing bocce ball, I could not believe who I spotted walking toward me. It was my Navajo Indian friend, Lawrence.

"What are you doing here?" I asked him, smiling wide with the pleasure of seeing a familiar face.

"We drove down to bring you your three-year token for sobriety."

I saw that he had two attractive women with him. It dawned on me that the three of them had driven at least four hours to see me. We hugged each other, and he gave me the bronze token commemorating my three years of sobriety. The Roman numeral III appeared on one side, and The Serenity Prayer was inscribed on the other. I was so grateful that Lawrence came to see me, even though I was embarrassed to be at a psychiatric hospital.

Occupational therapy usually consisted of guided exercises with art work, mostly pencil-paper activities, sometimes water color, and sometimes magic markers. All the activities centered on emotions, but I attempted to remain fairly quiet about my emotions. Once I drew a large red scribble of anger and colored it with several shades of red, furiously working the crayons down almost to the last piece. Fortunately for me, we ran out of time before I was asked to talk about my feelings. I certainly knew I was quite angry, but what was the focus? Was I angry at the many professionals who could not help me? Was I angry because I felt like the butt of a cruel joke God played on me? Was I angry with some of my relatives or with the scuba diving instructor? No, I think I was most angry with myself—I still blamed myself for making a mistake during the dive and not following up immediately.

11
THE DRAMA CONTINUES

My ordeal in the hospital, hellish though it was, educated me about certain realities. For example, until we began hearing about traumatic brain injuries suffered by vast numbers of soldiers serving in Afghanistan and Iraq, I believe most Americans were in the dark about the consequences of brain injury. Perhaps many citizens still are. But during my group therapy sessions, I met a woman who had fallen from the edge of a waterfall and suffered brain damage. Unlike me, whose injury led me to be as quiet as possible, this woman's injury caused her to talk constantly. Sadly, everyone tried to stay away from her, for fear of being trapped by her incessant chatter.

I met another young man whose brain had been damaged in an automobile accident. I recall that he was a great Elvis impersonator, for all the good it did him. He had already been in and out of the state mental hospital facilities. Since I had almost wound up there myself, I asked him what it was like. He said that for sure, he no longer wanted to be warehoused in state hospitals. In fact, he enjoyed, as much as one can given the circumstances, being at this particular private mental facility. When I think back now, I realize that both these brain-injured individuals were considered locked in their conditions and not expected to get better. Their future involved nothing other than more mental facilities, public or private. Meanwhile, I logically tried to work my way toward suicide as the solution—there could be no other way. My main concern was not botching the job.

The group therapy sessions focused on relationships. One woman in particular stood out, because she was older and struggling with dementia. Yet because of the drugs she was taking, her mood was quite happy most of the time. She gave me a special prayer on a card—a novena. I copied that prayer by hand on the inside cover of my meditation book. Maria often sang for the group, but since the only song she knew was *You Are My Sunshine*, she became one more thing to steadily wear me down. My coping mechanism in group therapy involved turning off and tuning out, but nodding along as if I was paying attention.

One Sunday, Lyle and Nadine Houk came to the hospital and took me with them to church and then out to eat. Lyle had worked with my father at the New Mexico State Department of Agriculture, and they had been friends for as long as I could remember. I felt grateful for and uplifted by Lyle and Nadine's kindness in letting me escape from the routine at the hospital, even if only for part of a day. For those hours, I felt renewed optimism, as if all eventually would be right with the world.

I had been told that this hospital used psychodrama as a therapeutic tool, and despite my ongoing preoccupation with suicide, I believe it helped me the most emotionally. We met in the drama room, which had all sorts of optional props like foam bats, clothes, costumes, and chairs, and acted out an emotional problem that affected our lives. I watched for several days as the others worked through extremely emotional and painful tragedies in their lives. I sat in silence, but this activity had my attention.

One man in the group had lost his son and daughter-in-law to a drunk driver. Not long after this tragedy, he started hanging around bars late at night awaiting drunks as they left to get in their cars. He then attacked them and beat them up in order to take away their car keys. He was in deep legal trouble, although he had not killed anyone. More important, though, he was in serious trouble with himself. He'd been unable to forgive and move on. He took the foam rubber bat and beat the demons of his life right in front of us, and then he broke down and sobbed. This powerful psychodrama released a spirit of surrender in him, and I felt sure he'd been transformed by the activity.

Would I be able to release such emotion, freeing myself from my troubles? When my turn came in the psychodrama, I hoped for a miracle. I had been thinking long and hard about what issue I'd deal with, and I chose certain family members who I believed had betrayed me. They'd not been supportive during my recovery from alcoholism, and after my diving accident, they'd been quick to judge that I was, indeed, mentally ill.

The drama coach had me set out five empty chairs in the middle of the room. I could have asked other patients to sit in those chairs, but I chose to leave them empty. Had I placed real people in the chairs, I'd have had trouble focusing on the specific relatives in question. I really wanted to come to grips with my anger toward them.

I stood across from the carefully arranged chairs and envisioned my relatives sitting on them. I had a brief talk with each one, and then I dismissed them from my life. I didn't wish them any ill will, but I wanted them out of my life, at least for a while. I especially didn't want any more ill-advised medical advice from them. During this session, I didn't cry or swear, but sent them away from me and off to some safe place. After the exercise, I realized I'd experienced a degree of relief.

My relief was short lived as I got more depressing news. Now, even Dr. Butz argued that I did not have caisson disease (an older term for decompression illness). He called me to his office, and once there, I asked him about my decompression illness.

"Mr. Greathouse, you do not have caisson disease!" he yelled right in my face.

It was as if he took a knife and cut out the front portion of my brain. I went numb. How could I survive in a mental hospital if no one believed that I had the illness that I was convinced I had? Again, my world turned upside down. I became more convinced that death was my only escape. In fact, I felt as if Dr. Butz' arrogance had killed me.

"But what about my slurred speech and balance problems?" I argued back. I rarely questioned anyone during the long ordeal of misdiagnoses. However, this was the final battle line, although I knew I'd lose the battle. A damaged brain had little chance against a doctor of psychiatry.

Using Freudian terminology, the doctor explained that people can first believe they are paralyzed and then actually become paralyzed with no medical cause. He believed that I was such a person. In other words, I *believed* that I had neurological symptoms of caisson disease, but no medical documentation supported this. This was difficult to argue against, because the CAT scans and MRIs hadn't turned up anything to substantiate brain damage from decompression illness. Naturally, given my fragile state, I wondered if I literally had thought myself into this condition. In the face of this authority figure, I doubted everything.

During this time, I called my parents, but had little good to say. I know I sounded extremely ungrateful for what they'd done to get me out of jail and into this safe facility. I was preoccupied with thoughts of getting my brain back. "Professionals" locked me down, jailed me, drugged me, and talked to me, but no one could cure me. Each time I called my parents, I upset them more, so I vowed not to call them. I knew little of their emotional turmoil or their resolve not to give up on me. Just when I thought all was lost, they were continuing the battle behind the scenes.

In fact, my father had become even more serious about finding help. I was unaware of his actions, but through ongoing contact with a variety of people, he got his hands on information about delayed treatment for decompression illness. This led him to contact the Undersea and Hyperbaric Medical Society in Bethesda, Maryland. My father is a key behind-the-scenes hero in this story, but my own confusion limited my understanding of my father's efforts on my behalf.

It would take many more pages to fully relate the series of phone calls and contacts that took place to various doctors, including Paul Harch in New Orleans. I mention this because you, too, may be in a situation where it seems impossible to get help, or perhaps, you or your advocate may be tempted to give up. But it may be that one more phone call is what ultimately changes the situation for you or your loved one.

During the course of my father's search, he learned that Dr. Harch worked at JoEllen Smith Medical Center in New Orleans, Louisiana, specifically in the Department of Emergency and Hyperbaric Medicine. While talking with my father, Dr. Harch related that he worked with hyperbaric oxygen all the time, especially with the commercial divers on the oil platforms in the Gulf of Mexico. Although he had been unable to persuade the New Mexico HBOT doctors to provide adequate delayed treatments for me, he offered my father hope. He indicated that he believed my scuba diving accident most probably resulted in an air embolism and decompression illness and that delayed treatments might still help. Over the next several days, my father and Dr. Harch spoke by telephone many more times.

Meanwhile, back in the hospital, I fell into a severe depression. Various lab tests were done, and to the surprise of no one, I was diagnosed with clinical depression. This diagnosis led to talk of medication, which bothered me even more because I had been sober and substance free for three years. But I was told that I'd be given a new generation antidepressant manufactured in England—Anafronil, a tricyclic antidepressant. Despite reassurances, I feared a repeat of my Thorazine stupor, which I knew would finish me.

That evening, when the nurse dispensed medication from the window of the pharmacy area, she called my name. I reluctantly approached the window, where she gave me the medication in a small plastic container and handed me some water in a paper cup. She watched as I swallowed the pill.

I walked away in defeat. Later, I went into the game room and sat with a patient who was smoking a cigarette. For some reason, watching her smoke made me feel resigned to my condition in life. I hadn't smoked in years, but I thought, "What the heck, I might as well start smoking again, too." So, I asked her for a cigarette and she thrust the pack toward me. I smoked while I listened to her complain about her mental illness—bipolar disorder.

Unbeknownst to me, my mother had a key phone conversation with Dr. Harch. Now, so many years later, Dr. Harch and my mother have helped me reconstruct the gist of this conversation. Dr. Harch wanted to know details of my earlier, three-treatment experience with HBOT. Specifically, had the doctors in New Mexico followed his prescribed protocol (they hadn't) and what were the results? My mother brought him up to date, recounting the unbelievable chain of events, including my time in jail and my current incarceration in the psychiatric hospital.

Dr. Harch had told the doctors about a diver he'd treated the year before, and he'd encouraged them to try the same thing at the New Mexico facility. Dr. Harch absolutely believed I had brain decompression illness—that's all there was to it. He could see no reason why the same treatment protocol wouldn't help me. At the same time, Dr. Harch hoped that my mother would *ask* him to take my case. You see, he was reluctant to say, "Drag him out of the psych hospital against the judge's orders and bring him to me. I'll treat him."

However, near the end of the conversation, my mother blurted, "Well, Dr. Harch, will you take his case?"

Dr. Harch replied, "I thought you would never ask."

Around this time, I learned I was scheduled for release from the psych hospital just in time for me to return to my junior high school math teaching position. Huh? How could I continue teaching math when I could no longer accurately count or write legibly on the chalkboard? I stumbled and slurred my words. Anafronil was not a miraculous cure that made me normal again. No way could I continue teaching.

Sometimes, a sense of calm would gently overtake me, and I could sit for hours slowly putting pieces of a jigsaw puzzle together. Then my calm bubble would burst when one of the staff members challenged me about wasting my time working on the puzzles. I had no way to defend myself or explain why I preferred to sit quietly and fit pieces by trial and error, along with some limited cognitive visual matching of colors and themes. This is what I felt capable of doing.

Quite often, the puzzles featured classic scenes of snowy, rural New England. This scenery still fascinates me. I can close my eyes, letting my current redeemed and productive life recede, and I see jigsaw puzzle pieces forming the snowy landscape, the tracks through the road, the snow-laden branches of the wooded farm scene, and the golden touches of the slowly sinking sun. The dark purples, the brilliant whites, and the golden rays of that place somewhere in New England still call to me so many years later. At the time, the magnetism of the jigsaw puzzles held a bit of hope. The pastoral scenes beckoned me to jump inside them and escape my dismal existence.

One evening I had a nice surprise—an unexpected break in my trance—when a good high school friend, who taught in Albuquerque, came by to visit me. A pleasant Christian woman, Connie had found out that I was in the hospital. Although I could have refused to see her, I decided against blocking her visit. She brought some games and several patients settled around a table and began to play. I looked on and went through the motions, wondering if she could detect that I was drugged up pretty good, although it was nothing like the Thorazine stupor. The Anafronil trance was different in its effect and allowed me to be aware of Connie and the games, but not fully engaged.

While I remained unaware of it, my parents had made hotel reservations in Gretna, Louisiana, and I was scheduled for release from the hospital sometime near the end of August. Presumably, this coincided with the beginning of the school year. However, the real reasons for my early release were more complex. Dr. Harch had asked my mother to approach the district attorney to reconsider my commitment to the hospital. Since the judge had committed me, the district attorney was not going to allow my release without a good reason. Dr. Harch spoke with the district attorney. "Look," he said, "I believe that Dan has decompression illness. He can be helped, and I will be responsible for bringing him to New Orleans."

I didn't know I was leaving the hospital until my mother picked me up and helped me gather my things. I recall that Mom was agitated after meeting with Dr. Butz, but in my haze, I knew only that the two disagreed about something important. Later, I learned that Dr. Butz warned my mother that she'd be traveling 1000 miles only to waste her money and resources on some quack.

I also recall asking my mother what she thought about my ability to teach.

"Hell no, you can't teach," she replied, "but you are not going back to work anyway, because we are taking you to Dr. Harch in New Orleans."

I had trouble processing what I'd just heard. "Did you say we were going to New Orleans?"

"Yes, your father and I have made arrangements for you to meet Dr. Harch. We are going to try to help you."

"It's too late," I protested. "I should have been treated a long time ago. There is no way I can be helped now." I said all that because I didn't want to get my hopes up too much. Yet, I didn't want to dampen her determination, as if I could have done such a thing. My mother is a very determined woman!

Given all that had happened, I still find it astounding to recall how many doctors openly referred to Dr. Harch as a quack. Every time my mother or I mentioned his name, the doctors spouted judgments about him. They had never once discussed the science of HBOT or probed into the stories of other divers treated with HBOT. Years later, I remain perplexed by not only the quick judgments about Dr. Harch, but also the level of ignorance and lack of curiosity about hyperbaric medicine on the part of so many medical professionals.

With my father and brother sharing legs of the driving, we headed for New Orleans. I was uncommunicative and confused much of the time, but eventually I woke to see the morning sun splattering its dappled light within the shadows of the old city square in Opelousas, once the capital of Louisiana. Opelousas? I thought I was really losing my mind when we stopped in this town. I had never heard of such a place. Was this a dream or reality? When one of the town markers indicated that it had once been the capital of Louisiana, I knew I was losing my mind. The mind, even my damaged one, has a fascinating ability to remember such trivia. It was only years later while writing this book, that I researched this town some and found out that it actually was the capital of Louisiana for nine months after Baton Rouge fell to the Union army during the Civil War in 1862. We had driven over long stretches of farmland near antebellum mansions camouflaged by Spanish moss dangling from the branches of live oaks.

Earlier, thick morning fog prohibited a clear view of these mansions, but they stood mysteriously in the mist.

It is funny how some quirky word or thing is so remembered in the midst of the fog of brain injury. Usually it would be some insignificant piece of trivia and almost never an important piece of information. I would often learn a new word and ruminate and obsess on that particular word for days, sometimes weeks. Opelousas ran round and round in my mind, and I wondered who ever came up with such a word as "Opelousas"? I felt as if I could ward off brain damage by magically learning some odd, trivial piece of information to impress people around me, so they would say there was certainly nothing wrong with a person who could memorize such an important fact about Opelousas as being a former state capital of Louisiana.

The silence of the smooth asphalt ride blended surrealistically with the inner calm of my heart that morning. It wouldn't be long before we'd arrive in New Orleans. Still, I was acutely aware that I was no longer the Dan Greathouse I knew. The old Dan could think quickly, read without losing his place, and add numbers together in his mind. And he could easily count the number of columns on the portico of any Southern mansion without losing his place.

But in my wildest dreams I *never* could have imagined what would happen in New Orleans.

12
"THE FOLKS FROM NEW MEXICO ARE HERE"

Memory is a strange faculty, and we never know what each of us will remember about certain events in life. I do recall that as we drove along, I was no longer as agitated about my condition. The antidepressants provided "the serenity to accept the things I could not change" in pill form. A change of scene didn't hurt either, and I allowed myself to hope.

As we neared New Orleans, I noted all the water in the bayous and how green the plant life was. I could almost smell the frogs and slithery swamp life that I imagined thrived in such places. We'd entered a new world, over 1000 miles away from home, and when I could concentrate, it fascinated me.

Once in New Orleans, we made our way to the La Quinta Inn in Gretna. Later that day, Dad talked with Dr. Harch, who outlined the tentative schedule for the next day. I was extremely tired from the trip, but my father and brother decided to explore the area. When they'd left, I crawled up onto the nice soft bed and turned on the television to settle back and watch an old black and white classic movie. I was asleep within minutes.

I mark August 29, 1991, as one of the most important days in my life, because it was the first day I visited the JoEllen Smith Emergency and Hyperbaric Medicine Unit. The sun shone brightly on the light colored bricks of the building, but I recall most vividly the paralyzing heat and humidity. I had never felt anything quite like this boiling, suffocating heat, not even on my trip to Cancun, Mexico.

As we walked through the building, we turned a corner and saw a huge room with an odd-looking piece of equipment—it reminded me of an airplane fuselage. It turned out to be a multi-place hyperbaric chamber unit, with an enormous number of pipes and gauges. Dad asked one of the blue-uniformed hyperbaric techs where we might meet Dr. Harch. The tech asked if we were the folks that had driven all the way from New Mexico. My father told him that we were, indeed, those folks.

The technician picked up the phone to call Dr. Harch and asked, "Would there be some folks that drove all the way from New Mexico to see you about a scuba diving accident?"

This technician was unaware that arrangements had already been made, but he thought it odd that anyone from the dry state of New Mexico would travel such a distance to see Dr. Harch about a scuba diving accident. Years later, Dr. Harch recalled this moment as one of our lighter ones in New

Orleans.

When Dr. Harch came into the unit and approached us, I was surprised to see a man who appeared to be somewhat younger than me. I immediately noticed his great enthusiastic spirit and bright eyes—I sensed brilliant intelligence behind those eyes. I stumbled toward him and said, "They say you might be able to help me." I slurred my speech, but I managed not to lose my balance altogether.

Dr. Harch assured me he was going to run some tests to determine if I had decompression illness. Attentive and compassionate, he asked me about the scuba diving accident, and I did my best to relate all that had happened.

At some point, my father and brother left the examination room, and Dr. Harch continued interviewing and examining me. He had me stand up and close my eyes. Then I was to walk in place, keeping my arm pointed in the same direction. When he asked me to open my eyes, I was pointing in an entirely different direction. My proprioceptive abilities were clearly impaired. For all my balance problems, I'd not been aware of that one before that day.

Looking back, I can only imagine the pressure Dr. Harch faced in trying to determine if I was mentally ill or if I actually had central nervous system decompression illness. Later, Dr. Harch told my father that he needed to conduct several tests over the next couple of days. Before we left that first day, I turned to Dr. Harch and in a pleading tone said, *"Doc, I want my brain back."*

The next day, I met with Dr. Mendoza, a psychologist, and spent several hours in his office answering questions and performing various tasks. He also gave me a lengthy personality inventory to complete and return to him in a couple of days. After the morning session, I had an appointment with an ear, nose, and throat specialist for an ENG test, the same one I'd done with Dr. Thorne back in New Mexico, two months earlier. After I had a hearing test, I realized it was my third auditory evaluation. Once again, all the testing made me feel like a zombie. I met with another doctor for neuropsychological tests, including several memory subtests. I didn't like those tests, because my memory was more or less gone. But I cooperated because Dr. Harch needed them.

Dr. Mendoza was a pleasant man with a gentle spirit about him. This helped me greatly, because I was feeling the pressure of being ushered to so many tests. I even visited another neurologist and had another CAT scan. I hadn't experienced this much activity in a very long time, so I ended up extremely exhausted at the end of each day. Fortunately, my father and brother were there to drive me all over New Orleans for the various tests.

During down time, Dad and Ross often dragged me out of the dark hotel room. The bright light of day always stabbed deeply into my eyes, and I preferred to go back to hiding in the dark. On one trip, we drove across the

Lake Pontchartrain Causeway to the North Shore. The reason this trip stands out is that we saw several young men dressed as clowns inside a small VW Bug with a sunroof. One clown rode with his head stuck out of the top, and his multicolored rainbow clown wig shone bright in the sun. His white-washed face with the perpetual smile intrigued me—I wanted to trade places with him. I felt merely one step away from being a clown myself.

I thought about being a silent clown who went into hospitals to cheer up terminally ill children. I wouldn't need to know cute jokes or stories to distribute candy or coloring books to these children. I would sport a traditional white painted face with accentuated red lips and exaggerated eyelashes and eyebrows. I could imagine being crowned with some god-awful huge orange bush for hair, no bald head for me, thank you. Checkered black and white torn pants and large pontoon-sized shoes would fit nicely. Of course, I worried about how I might walk with such exaggerated foot extension, but it wouldn't matter. The children would laugh. They would laugh all they wanted. I would have fulfilled my purpose to cheer them up.

On another trip, I went with Dad and Ross to the Aquarium of the Americas. Although I remember very little about it, I do recall that in the tropical plant section I almost fell over when a bird squawked as it flew across my path. I didn't handle unexpected noises or movements very well. Things that would have been marvelous adventures at one time in my life were too much for me. Oh, how I envied my father and brother for being able to enjoy the sightseeing so much.

Old fears arose as the days passed. What if I went through all these tests, some for the second and third time, only to learn nothing could be done for me? It was so difficult to keep the faith, although I knew that other people carried me with their prayers. Because I had to go off the antidepressant meds in order to repeat the ENG test, my mood worsened.

The day I had to go to an imaging center, I became more agitated than usual, protesting that I'd had MRIs before, so why should I have another? The dark confines of the MRI machine tube bothered me, and besides, I was convinced the test would discover nothing new. As the medication wore off, I realized how drugged I'd been. But at the same time, I'd become more despondent and subject to outbursts of anger. I began swearing again and taking my moods out on Dad and Ross, behavior that again made me a serious burden.

One afternoon, I staggered over to the nearby gas station and bought a pack of cigarettes. I had quit smoking just before beginning my trip to New Orleans, because I had hope for life once again. I had put the cigarettes down without a second thought. But, without the medication, I was again overwhelmed and hopeless. I sat on the steps of the hotel and smoked while Dad and Ross were inside. It was now almost four months since the scuba diving accident at Lake Powell and weeks since I'd been to my spiritual support group meetings. Dad and Ross provided consistent support in many respects, but I didn't feel comfortable sharing with them. Besides, I had become a broken record, saying the same things over and over about how I had brain damage and how worried I was. I was truly self-absorbed.

The next thing I remember was going back into the room, all the while ranting, raving, cursing, and slamming my fists into the door. Dad and Ross were completely shocked, as they had not seen this behavior in quite some time. The medication had worked to calm me, but now my frustration and outbursts were back. Dad tried to call Dr. Harch, but reached another doctor who advised him to bring me into the Department of Emergency and Hyperbaric Medicine.

Dad and Ross drove me to the emergency room where I was given Valium. Even in my despondent mental state, they were going to perform yet another test while they had me there; an "evoked potential brain stem study," which had also been done in New Mexico. The Valium provided a sweet comfort that blanketed my body in peace. As I relaxed on the gurney, I no longer cared that I would have another test—they could have performed medical tests all night long as far as I was concerned. I drifted into near sleep as the medical staff attached electrodes to my head and calibrated the machines, while various colored lights blinked in the dimly lit room.

That evening, I went to the JoEllen Smith Psychiatric Hospital. I walked toward the entrance of an attractive building surrounded by beautiful green trees, shrubs, and flowering plants, and with many large windows. It was evening, and the sunset was brilliant with bright orange, gold, and yellow splashing on the clouds. This was like beginning some new golden age of my life. Valium-induced serenity was a wonderful thing.

I was admitted to the chemical dependency unit, rather than the psychiatric unit, in order to monitor my withdrawal from Anafronil. Dr. Harch later commented that I'd crashed so hard from the withdrawal that I'd become catatonic. In other words, I had reached a point of psychomotor retardation; I was literally so depressed that I could not move. He described me as "sitting on the bunk bed in a stupor." Despite this setback, Dr. Harch wanted to confirm my diagnosis of brain decompression illness, and said a SPECT blood flow scan would help with this confirmation.

Dr. Harch likes to obtain before and after scans to document the changes in the brain. SPECT stands for "Single Photon Emission Computed Tomography," and it differs from PET, which stands for "Positron Emission Tomography," in that it's a high resolution form of functional brain imaging. At the time, next to PET, SPECT was one of the best ways to look at brain function. A high resolution SPECT scan uses a triple-headed camera, meaning the three cameras on the machine obtain a high resolution, three-dimensional representation of blood flow in the brain.

Although I'd already had other brain imaging tests that appeared normal, Dr. Harch said they couldn't possibly be entirely accurate since I was unable to walk in a straight line, not to mention all my other problems. After the baseline SPECT brain scan was completed, the radiologist called Dr. Harch and told him he needed to look at the scan. He said, "something was really wrong in this guy's brain." Dr. Harch would find the results to be as dramatic as the radiologist had indicated.

During my stay at JoEllen Smith Psychiatric Hospital, I noted that the staff had nothing but good things to say about Dr. Harch, which made my confidence in him grow. I also attended group therapy sessions, where—at last—I felt useful. Despite all that I had been through, I had not started drinking and still had my three years of sobriety. "They always said to just not drink no matter what, even if my bottom were to fall off," I shared. I told them about my scuba diving accident and why I had come to New Orleans—troubled, going through withdrawal, but still sober.

Dr. Harch ordered many more medical tests during the next ten days and had me transported by ambulance all over New Orleans for the various assessments. One particular test involved endoscopy (sending an exploratory tube down the esophagus) and was meant to provide information about my heart and lungs using a type of sonic wave imagery. Once the procedure began, the doctors became quite excited about discovering something of scientific note about the passage of air bubbles from one chamber of my heart to another. I did not fully understand what happened, but when air was injected to be monitored, there was an unexplained, and before this time, undocumented, transference of air bubbles between the chambers of my heart. Later, Dr. Harch referred to this phenomenon as the "Greathouse effect." He also reminded me that this was actually air bubbles passing through the lungs. Because of this physiological anomaly, I had a greater potential for air bubbles to reach the brain, which contributed to my decompression sickness. Dr. Harch also wanted one more test, the rotary chair test, which assesses balance. I had done poorly on it back in New Mexico three months earlier and didn't do well this time either.

One evening, Dr. Harch and Dr. Adrian Blotner, my psychiatrist at the unit, came to visit me and suggested that I begin taking a relatively low dose of Prozac, just as a short-term intervention. Dr. Harch explained that we had a window of opportunity in which the Prozac would stimulate my neural connections, while my brain was making new connections as a result of the HBOT.

Within a few days, Dr. Harch confirmed to my father that I did indeed have decompression illness, a belief he'd had even prior to the SPECT scan. However, the SPECT brain scans documented the decompression illness in such a way that he could demonstrate this to other doctors. By using before and after scans, he could show improvement from the treatment. Dr Harch also issued a statement, which my father and I found profound, because it at last made sense of all I'd been through—and it changed the course of my life. It reads as follows:

Mr. Greathouse is under the care of myself and a team of specialists at the Jo Ellen Smith Medical Center Hyperbaric Medicine and Diving Unit in New Orleans, Louisiana, for evaluation and treatment of central nervous system decompression sickness experienced during a diving accident May 19, 1991, at Lake Powell, Arizona. Due to the nature of his illness and the necessity for extended neuro rehabilitation, Mr. Greathouse will be unable to resume teaching duties for a minimum of six to eight weeks. During this time he will be residing in New Orleans for neuro rehabilitation and prolonged hyperbaric oxygen therapy. We will keep you apprised at the next interval, in approximately six weeks, of his progress and ability to return to work. If you have any questions we can be reached at the Hyperbaric Medicine and Diving Unit.

Dr. Harch had put in writing what he'd believed all along. Prior to the SPECT scan, he had decided to treat me regardless of whether or not he could confirm it, because he thought we had nothing to lose. His initial belief about my illness was based on everything he had heard regarding my condition combined with what he knew about HBOT and its effect on the body. Now, with the brain scans, he had undeniable scientific proof. He was particularly interested to see if I would show improvement like the other diver whom he had successfully treated the year before.

Dr. Harch's words also confirmed that I was not a hopeless case, which brought me both relief and joy. Even if the treatments didn't work, I had a diagnosis that made sense. And I wasn't crazy.

Before we came to New Orleans, Dr. Harch had told my mother about successfully treating a diver the year before. This patient had also been considered demented—in fact, he was about to become a story on the evening news. Dr. Harch treated him with hyperbaric oxygen therapy, and he improved substantially. The treatment took place seven to eight months after his decompression illness accident, which represented a breakthrough in treatment and went against conventional wisdom. The issue has been controversial in medicine and neurology, not because anyone questions HBOT's usefulness in treating decompression illness in divers immediately following a diving accident, but rather, because many question the efficacy of *delayed* treatment. The diving medicine "establishment" has said no, but pioneering HBOT specialists, like Dr. Harch, believe otherwise.

At the time, this didn't make an impression on me, because my memory was bad and I was doing so poorly myself. But later, I was able to fill in the picture and understand how much I benefitted from Dr. Harch's experience with the other diver's case.

Later on the same day that Dr. Harch officially provided my diagnosis in a written statement, one of the young men in the chemical dependency unit celebrated thirty days of being clean from drugs, and his family showed up with food—delicious Louisiana dishes. Although I hadn't touched a piano in several months, I couldn't resist sitting down at the piano in the day room. I attempted to play *In the Mood*, and enjoyed myself, mistakes and all. I laughed with the others and had a good time.

The next morning, after my ten days of hospitalization, I was released from JoEllen Smith and returned to stay at the La Quinta Inn. Nathan, an old friend of my dad's, had come to New Orleans to be with him after my brother went home. My parents needed their support systems, too. Since Dad had to fly home, Nathan carefully explained the yellow highlighted route from the hotel to the Hyperbaric Medicine Diving Unit. I wasn't sure about driving myself, but Dad insisted that I'd be okay on my own in New Orleans. I guess he had more faith in my driving abilities than I did.

The La Quinta Inn itself was convenient and had gracious managers who made us feel welcome. A restaurant and mall were within walking distance, and much to my surprise, other than the driving issue, I wasn't too worried about being on my own. My excitement about treatment proved to be stronger than my fears.

Before Nathan and Dad went home, they took me on a riverboat ride. The day was warm and bright. Finally, my mood was good enough, even without medication, to enjoy seeing the river and the backwoods bayou country. I'd reached a new point in my journey, where my hope had come to something, rather than the dead ends of the previous months. Hope is an amazing and powerful thing. We can lose everything in the world, but if we hold on to hope, the human spirit can endure any hardship. I was glad to have hope in my life again. I had no idea if the HBOT would be successful, and Dr. Harch had made no promises. But, between the two of us, we had hope that I would get better.

13
THE MIRACLE IN NEW ORLEANS

While I was on the boat tour with Dad and his friend, Nathan, I heard beautiful calliope music coming from a huge paddlewheel boat. I dared not dream of being able to play music again, but I could enjoy the music and revel in the fact that at least for that one day I had rediscovered hope. The weather was oppressively hot, but I didn't even seem to mind the heat so much anymore. After the boat trip, the three of us walked along the waterfront taking in the sights. Then Dad and Nathan took me to a barbershop where I had my hair cut short and my beard shaved off. There! I'd spruced up for the next phase of my recovery. Cure or no cure, I looked a little more civilized. In this heat, I was cooler, too, without a beard.

Finally, the time came for Dad and Nathan to leave the car with me and fly back home. That meant driving back to the hotel from the airport alone. I tried to remain fairly calm about the prospect of navigating the big, white 1988 Oldsmobile through the maze and confusion of New Orleans traffic—and not weave too much! Luckily, their flight wasn't scheduled during rush hour. While Nathan assured my father that I'd be fine, he might not have sounded so confident if he'd known how hard I was working to hide my nervousness.

I found I was no longer depressed about my condition. And, I'd learned that two other commercial divers living at the La Quinta Inn also were taking hyperbaric oxygen therapy under the supervision of Dr. Harch. During my stay at the JoEllen Smith Psychiatric Hospital, both my father and brother had told me about a commercial diver, only nineteen years old, who'd had a diving accident while working on an oil platform in the Gulf of Mexico. He had not been decompressed correctly, and his sickness resulted in paralysis from the waist down—he had no feeling whatsoever. HBOT had helped him to walk again, although he still had no sensation in his hips, legs, or feet. His story had the ring of a miracle, since I'd never heard of any paralyzed person being able to walk again, unless the cause had been psychological in the first place.

Despite the fact that I was going to be alone in New Orleans and had not seen any improvement in my neurological deficits, I found that my fear was gone along with my suicidal thoughts. Obtaining a correct diagnosis had done wonders for me. I no longer faced psychiatrists and group therapy or jail. The new scientific approach I'd embarked on made all those other strategies, even modern psychiatry, seem like little more than medieval cures based on superstition.

I'd reached a point at which I didn't know if HBOT would cure me, but no matter what, I wouldn't have to go through life wondering about my diagnosis. I finally had an answer to silence the many armchair psychologists who were a "little more than kin and a little less than kind."

As Dad and Nathan prepared to leave for the airport, I mentally rehearsed my way back to the hotel and attempted to remain calm. Fortunately, the Prozac, which I was taking on a gradual build-up dosage level, allowed me to stay alert, rather than giving me the zombie-like feeling I'd had while on Anafronil. Only a couple of months earlier, no one in my family would have allowed me to be alone for fear that I might kill myself. We truly had come a long way already.

Dad drove to the airport, while Nathan reviewed the different landmarks and eased my mind about the trip back. I felt like a young child being sent to school by myself for the first day. Dad and Nathan were the loved ones filling me in on the rules, and making sure I knew how to find my way back home without talking to strangers or becoming lost in a maze of side streets and alleys.

After we said our goodbyes at the airport, I watched the plane take off with the only two people I had known in New Orleans. But I was excited, too, about finding my way through the city. Nathan's directions and good coaching paid off, and I had no problem getting back to the hotel—even in time for lunch.

Just outside my hotel room, a muscular man with a shaved head approached me. In a voice scratchy from too many cigarettes, he asked if I was Dan Greathouse.

I introduced myself and he told me his name was Rod, one of the two divers receiving HBOT. I couldn't help but be excited to meet another person with decompression sickness. As it turned out, Dr. Harch had talked about me and my situation. I immediately felt a kinship with Rod, and he was most informative and enthusiastic about the hyperbaric oxygen treatments that were helping him.

Rod's story was different from mine in that he'd been decompressed incorrectly. Apparently, the person running the chamber had not sealed the door correctly, resulting in Rod getting "a hit." He explained that decompression illness hits different people in different places, and his hit was in his shoulder where he was experiencing osteonecrosis—or dying bone tissue.

We talked for a long time and then went out for lunch, where we talked even more. I listened intently to every word Rod had to share about the treatment program, and he answered all my questions.

"These people are angels, I tell you, Greathouse," Rod said at one point. "They have really helped quite a few divers. Everything that happens over in those chambers is like a miracle."

That's exactly what I wanted and needed to hear. For the next couple of hours, Rod described the grueling work done by commercial divers on the oil platforms in the Gulf of Mexico. He also talked about how they often were pushed beyond reasonable limits. Sure, the pay was good, but the risk was high, too, and the accidents weren't necessarily the fault of the divers. Rod also mentioned that substance abuse was common on these rigs, and sometimes the workers in charge of the decompression chambers were too drunk or high to run them competently. He described situations in which the operators placed the divers in the chambers, but then haphazardly adjusted the settings while drifting about in the fog of their altered state. They only went through the motions and collected a paycheck. The workload was extremely demanding, and when a crew came ashore the parties were endless. (I have no personal knowledge of the conditions about which Rod spoke, so I'm simply repeating his descriptions.)

I found Rod's stories fascinating, but the best part was my relief in meeting a real person who suffered from decompression illness. Before speaking with Rod, I'd learned everything I knew about decompression illness from *The MERCK Manual* and my diving instruction lesson book.

Rod assured me that I'd be helped. "Just wait and see, Greathouse," he said. He also talked about the young paralyzed man, Mitch. Rod believed that Dr. Harch and his associates had worked a miracle on Mitch, even though his symptoms hadn't completely reversed, and he lacked feeling in half his body. Mitch had made progress, though, in that he started out unable to walk and had improved to using a walker and then a cane. Yet, his motor problems had started out worse than mine.

After lunch Rod and I started back to the hotel, where I'd have a chance to meet Mitch. My relief in not feeling so alone overwhelmed me, and tears of joy built in the corners of my eyes. I once again felt so grateful that my parents and Ross hadn't given up on me.

Once at the hotel, I went to Rod and Mitch's room. Mitch looked so young sitting on the edge of his bed playing a video game. He barely acknowledged me, but I was just glad to meet him.

He finally spoke, "So you the Scooby doer from New Mexico?"

"Scooby doers are how we refer to sports divers," Rod said with a laugh.

"Yes, that would be me," I said.

Mitch said he was from New Mexico, too, but remained focused on the video game, never once looking up to make eye contact with me. That was okay, because I was extremely tired and needed to go back to my room. Once there, I fell fast asleep, waking up completely disorientated, but not frightened, in the middle of the night.

At the time, I didn't know that Dr. Harch had assured my parents that he was going to treat me regardless of what happened with the tests or the insurance company issues. He had decided to treat me at the facility he owned, because he could better control the cost. He was even ready to treat me for free if needed. He had decided to give me eighty hyperbaric treatments, because that number had worked on the previous diver, and he wanted to replicate the treatment so over time he could establish a protocol.

Early the next morning, I was awakened with a phone call indicating a taxi was waiting for me. I wondered what that was all about. I hurriedly dressed and carefully stumbled down the stairs to the hotel lobby to grab a cup of coffee. Janice and Kenneth, the hotel managers, told me to hurry and that gave me a chance to ask about the taxi. Apparently, the taxi would pick me up every day and take me to the clinic.

This was news I liked, because it meant I didn't have to drive. Besides, I was going to a different location for treatments than I'd originally thought. Buddy, the driver, a very friendly sort of fellow, explained that either he or another cab driver would pick me up each day to take me to the Emergency Physicians Treatment Center. Dr. Harch had made the transportation arrangements, a much welcomed "no-brainer" for me.

Once in the one-storied brick building, I met Jana, a hyperbaric technician, and Wanda, a licensed nurse. Dr. Staab was the doctor on call that day. Wanda and Jana checked my vital signs and my ears, and gave me hospital scrubs to put on in the nearby dressing room. I also had to take off my watch. Although Dr. Harch said that very few accidents occurred in hyperbaric chambers, there could be no sparks of any kind inside the oxygen-filled enclosures.

The treatment room held five or six monoplace hyperbaric oxygen chambers just like the one in which I'd had three treatments in New Mexico, three months earlier. So, this is where I'd have eighty treatments, one in the morning and one in the afternoon, over the next forty days. I crawled up onto the sliding padded platform that would be my resting place for the next ninety minutes. Jana explained that I would need to equalize the pressure by popping my ears, a process I'd become familiar with during my earlier treatments.

Luckily, a television set was mounted up on the wall, which I could see through the clear chamber walls. For the next weeks, my morning ritual included TV shows like *Family Feud*, *Regis Philbin*, and *Designing Women*, programs I hadn't seen before. But I was content to watch them, while the oxygen made a hissing sound as it filled my chamber with the miraculous gas. Now and then Jana or Wanda would check on me by speaking into the microphone connected to the chamber, but we never really talked at great lengths during the sessions. The ninety minutes flew by, and then it was time for the attendants to lower the pressure in the chamber. My ears always popped the most during this portion of the treatment. Soon, I was out of the chamber and changing out of my scrubs and into my clothes.

After that first morning treatment, a van picked me up and took me to the Rehabilitation Institute of New Orleans, where I had an appointment with a physiatrist (rehabilitation physician) named Dr. Katz. He put me through my paces, literally. He had me walk heel to toe down the hallway amongst other tasks. That day I had a tour of the Rehabilitation Institute and was introduced to my physical therapist, speech/language therapist, and my socialization director.

Time flew by here, too. I ate lunch with the socialization director and several of the outpatients, which became part of my routine each weekday. I was exhausted, yet I still had an afternoon treatment scheduled. Once back at the hotel, I pulled the blinds closed to keep the bright sun out. Then I dozed with the television on until it was time to go back for the afternoon treatment. Luckily, I awakened before the front desk called to let me know the taxi had arrived.

During the afternoon session on that day and those that followed, I usually felt too drained to pay attention to whatever TV program Jana and Wanda had on, but I didn't sleep either. I lay there quietly watching television in a zombie-like stupor. My neurological deficits always became worse at the end of the day, and my first day of treatment was no different.

Although I couldn't feel it, the almost silent magic of oxygen started to work on my damaged brain and slowly and purposefully fed oxygen to "idling" neurons. I felt no different after the first two hyperbaric oxygen treatments, but I was completely exhausted. I barely remember the taxi ride back to the hotel, where I slept really well that afternoon and through the night.

The next morning, I had time to eat breakfast at Denny's before Buddy arrived to pick me up. I listened while he shared things about living in New Orleans. Buddy eventually asked me why I was there, so I told him about my diving accident, but I skipped the parts about being jailed and institutionalized. I didn't want to either frighten him or engage in lengthy explanations. He told me he'd been taxiing people back and forth for HBOT for quite some time now, mostly diabetics. That piqued my curiosity, but Buddy admitted that he didn't know anything about the treatment—he imagined "hyperbarics" had something to do with "barracks." I found it odd that someone whose living involved taking people to and from a treatment facility hadn't asked more about it or gone into the hyperbaric unit to have a look. At the same time, though, I'd never heard of hyperbaric oxygen being used to treat diabetics.

"How does it help diabetics?" I asked.

"It helps heal their wounds," he replied.

"No kidding," I said.

Today, I understand that a wound in the brain after a diving accident is not so different from a foot wound sustained by a diabetic person.

After Buddy dropped me off, I began the morning ritual that would continue for another thirty-nine days. At first, I had difficulty changing out of my clothes and into my scrubs. It seemed to take me a long time to undress, because I had to sit down so not to lose my balance which was still a nagging concern. Looking back, I realize I was somewhat unaware of the extent of my cognitive limitations, because I felt hazy so much of the time. But the balance issue was always apparent.

During the first week of treatments, I had a second SPECT scan. As soon as I finished my morning hyperbaric treatment, Dr. Harch actually took me directly to the same facility that had performed my first high resolution scan. Once there, I met Dr. Gottlieb, an associate of Dr. Harch. Technicians injected me with radioactive dye and quickly escorted me to the imaging device. I lay on the table as three gray panels moved close to my head, and the imaging took place. Then I was taken into another room to wait for the results.

When Dr. Gottlieb came to the room, he spoke in an excited tone.

"I think we can help you."

"That's great," I replied, although I had no idea what he meant, since I didn't feel different.

Later, Dr. Harch explained that he did not wish for me to view the images of my brain just yet. However, that evening back at the hotel, Rod told me all about it. He didn't actually see the scans, but he'd likely overheard a conversation about me and the results of the brain imaging.

"Well, Greathouse, you should have seen those pics. Your brain looked like Swiss cheese with all those holes in it," Rod said, laughing.

His words, or his levity, didn't bother me, perhaps because all along I'd known a spider had been inside my head gnawing on my brain tissue. Still, I'm glad that Dr. Harch had not shown me those pictures. He was wise not to. It was one thing for Rod to describe what he had seen or heard about, but it would have been an entirely different matter had I personally seen the imaging of my brain with holes.

I continued going to the Rehabilitation Institute every day where I participated in balance activities on low balance beams and worked with other devices designed to help rehabilitate people who had either suffered brain injury, spinal cord damage, or another kind of debilitating injury. I enjoyed the challenge of attempting to walk heel to toe, heel to toe, on a narrow wooden beam placed a few inches off the ground. At first, I couldn't keep my balance and fell off, but I kept trying. I also was introduced to a large wooden platform built on a pivot. I had to stand in the middle of the almost four by eight foot area and balance as if I were on a huge surfboard.

This platform was not only used for people who could walk, but it was also used for individuals who needed to learn to balance themselves in their wheelchairs.

This experience exposed me to people who were much more severely injured than I, which helped renew my gratitude. One day I saw a beautiful young woman attempting to walk with a newly attached artificial leg. She struggled and fell down, and then had to pull herself back up and start over again. I admired her determination, and she made a big impact on me.

One morning, Buddy picked me up and wanted to give me some Biblical literature, which I gladly accepted. I took the literature and read the Bible verses and annotations as well as I could. It was difficult at first to even try to concentrate, and I kept losing my place while reading, much like the way I lost focus on the TV programs during my treatments. I did try to memorize the names of the cast members on *Designing Women*, and each day I'd try to guess their names before it appeared on the screen next to their picture. This was my personal neuro-rehabilitation, along with the literature Buddy gave me.

I realized later that Buddy intended to get me to join his church, but he treated me kindly, so I didn't mind. In fact, he and his wife Jeri invited me to their church several times and even came by to pick me up. Once, they invited me to their house for a gathering where they served jambalaya and fillet gumbo. I will never forget their kindness to me. They became a kind of surrogate family, and Buddy continued to give me religious literature and even books. I could handle the pamphlets and small magazines, but I wasn't ready for the books—at least not yet.

14
IS THAT MY BRAIN TALKING TO ME?

If I hadn't experienced it myself, I would have found it difficult to believe that brain injuries could be treated with hyperbaric oxygen, or oxygen under pressure. Yet, as Dr. Harch reminds his patients, HBOT doesn't replace other neurological rehabilitation protocols or methods. For example, during my stay in New Orleans, I had a physical therapist, Teresa, with whom I worked on both an outdoor and indoor course. We used an intriguing computerized feedback machine, which determined if I was standing in balance without being on a balance beam.

I found the technology interesting, but I also had constant reminders of problems that lingered. On one particular day, I was embarrassed when Teresa had to tell me for about the fifth time to take my shoes off because they were making black marks on the workout mats. She'd told me to remove my shoes the first day, but I forgot the next, so she told me again, and then I forgot on the third day, and so it went for five days in a row. I kept forgetting, even though I wrote myself a reminder in my notebook. Not that Teresa was angry over it, but it embarrassed me that I could not think clearly enough to follow through.

At one point after the first full week of hyperbaric oxygen therapy, I got up in the middle of the night to relieve myself, and was pleasantly surprised to find that I was standing right there in the middle of the bathroom, not holding on to anything, without losing my balance. No weaving or bobbing about trying to keep from falling over. I was so excited that I never went back to sleep that night, but sat up writing in my journal about this extraordinary event. I even wrote a poem that I neatly copied, taking my time with it, too, because my fine motor skills were still not back.

The next day, I gave a copy of the poem to Jana and Wanda. My short poem spoke of them as angels performing miracles, but since they stayed so busy doing their routine work, they were likely unaware of the miracles happening because of their efforts. As you can guess, the return of my balance was an exciting miracle.

Of course, I had to call Mom and Dad to tell them the exciting news. This hyperbaric oxygen therapy was really working. I knew that only one week of physical rehabilitation could not bring about the return of my ability to balance. But the silent pressurized oxygen was doing its work to repair the blood flow in my brain, essentially switching on those parts that had been damaged during the diving accident. While amazed at this healing, I also noted that my back muscles were extremely sore. The muscles had compensated for my lack of balance for months, so in order to relax them, I needed extra physical therapy and heating compresses. Eventually, the muscles improved, but at first it felt as if an elephant had stepped on the middle of my back.

My twice a day treatments continued until midway through the treatment block, and then I had my third SPECT brain scan. I later learned that Dr. Harch ordered the extra scan because he'd observed that I wasn't making further improvement as I reached the thirty-five or forty treatment mark. Because I hadn't made additional gains during the last ten treatments, Dr. Gottlieb and Dr. Harch discussed the need to increase the dosage of hyperbaric oxygen. Upping the dosage would be facilitated by increasing the pressure. The new brain scan confirmed his suspicions, just as the first scan had confirmed his clinical suspicion of brain decompression illness. So, while I'd improved, the scan was still abnormal, and he decided to increase the dose of my hyperbaric oxygen and continue my treatment. Dr. Harch made it clear that he was not treating me solely based on the scan, but used the scan to help confirm the clinical signs.

About this time, a nurse made an offhand remark that left a seed of doubt in my mind. She spoke about HBOT as a great medical advance, but added, "If only it will last." This led to fears of regression, but Dr. Harch assured me this was not the case. In fact, when Dr. Harch called me at the Rehabilitation Institute during my socialization therapy, he explained that the "holes" in my imaging were about halfway filled in. That was a powerful and healing image.

Still, every now and then I'd get a sinking feeling that my story might turn out to be like *Flowers for Algernon,* where a patient makes great intellectual gains, but later regresses into mental retardation. Dr. Harch referred to my successful treatment as my "awakening." That called to mind the same image of miraculous healing depicted in the Robin William's movie *Awakenings,* which was also about improvement followed by regression. Eventually, though, I got past these fleeting fears.

Most of the time, the other patients in the hyperbaric unit were being treated for diabetic ulcers. However, a retired but famous lightweight champion boxer received treatments, too. Wanda told me he was being treated for years of sustained traumatic brain injury commonly referred to as being "punch drunk." I felt encouraged to see the doctors treating someone who obviously had sustained a brain injury earlier in life. I later asked Dr. Harch if the therapy had helped the boxer, and he said the boxer had become more aware of his mental status since receiving the therapy. Yes, he had received some benefit, but I am glad I did not wait as long as he had for therapy.

Alone in my hotel room one night, it suddenly hit me that I was thinking more. It was as if my brain consisted of a maze of corridors, and I was able to race about them in some shiny new sports car, whereas before I'd been trapped in slow motion thought processes. Some portions of my brain had been completely shut off by impenetrable doors. But now, I had the ability to think about one idea and then move to the next idea without laborious struggle. Each time I noticed an improvement, it was like someone had come along and flipped on a light switch in what had been a locked room.

Of course, I thought it was miraculous—magic—because I didn't know how hyperbaric oxygen therapy worked. In fact, scientists and clinicians like Dr. Harch and his colleagues were still determining the healing mechanism of HBOT. With my renewed thinking skills I began to wonder if HBOT could help friends of mine and other patients I'd just met at the Rehabilitation Institute. Most of all, I was ready to move the spider out of my brain, and I wanted to move back in.

I became a little more daring over time and attempted to drive the Oldsmobile into new areas of New Orleans, specifically the less congested parts. I wasn't ready for rush hour. But my thinking was still not clear, and one afternoon I attempted to refuel the car with diesel. Fortunately, the gas tank would not take the diesel nozzle, but I stood there and wondered what was wrong so that I couldn't make it fit. I've since been told I'm not the first person who absent-mindedly tried to fiddle around with the diesel nozzle before realizing they'd picked the wrong pump. And these individuals purportedly had all their mental capacities ticking right along. I also noticed that as the day grew longer, my abilities would still deteriorate somewhat. I had become used to this small fact of life, which is literally brain fatigue. This fatigue is rather ordinary, in that the cerebral cortex tires and the limbic brain can get the edge, which is why more fights and drinking and crime occur as the day wears on and turns into night. The rational part of the brain is tired and can't always overcome unwise emotional impulses.

Dr. Harch knew that I liked to play the piano, so he made arrangements for me to go to the nearby Aurora Country Club, where the manager, Joan Sokal, said I could practice on the piano during their slow hours in the middle of the afternoon. Excited about the chance to play, I found a music store where I bought a child's teaching book with simple classical pieces. Joan was quite pleasant and showed me to the piano, where I practiced for the next hour, which really tired me out. Dr. Harch commented that Joan thought I'd played well, but for some reason, I don't recall ever returning to the country club to practice. Maybe my rehabilitation schedule prevented me from going back. After all, I had two hyperbaric treatments a day, plus ongoing physical and speech/language therapy. Some evenings, I attended a Bible study with Buddy and Jeri. No wonder I slept so well during the nights.

The weekends were the slow time, although I still had hyperbaric treatments on both days. I'd meet with Rod and Mitch sometimes, but I never hung out with them, primarily because my commercial diver friends did a lot of smoking and drinking.

One day while in the chamber, another light switch came on. I could hear music in my head. I tapped my hands on the inside of the chamber while belting out, "I got a girl named Boney Maroney." The techs and the doctor came running out to check on me, but they laughed when they discovered I was celebrating the return of music to my head. Another miracle, another switch to the "on" position!

During this time I got out more and did things like go to the movies. One evening I called Brian, whom I had met at the Rehabilitation Institute. He had suffered traumatic brain injury from the violent actions of the hammer wielding drug addict who had attempted to kill him during a robbery. I offered to buy him dinner so we could talk about our brain injuries and about recovery. To meet him, I had to drive all the way through the busy part of New Orleans and across town to his address, but I was able to do so. We enjoyed some great food at the Algier's Landing Restaurant and watched the golden sunset to the west. We overheard other diners at a nearby table complain about small details and poor service. Brian and I laughed, because we had such a strong sense of appreciation for what we had, and we wouldn't have wasted time complaining about trivial things. After what we'd been through, we savored our restaurant food and the ability to even be there to enjoy it. It was wonderful to be alive.

During my time in New Orleans, summer turned into autumn. The days passed quickly, and soon my treatments would be completed. My physical abilities continued to improve, and I could stay on the balance beams longer and walk heel to toe without losing my balance. The therapists at the institute were quite amazed at how quickly I had recovered. I have no doubt that the hyperbaric oxygen therapy was the primary reason for such rapid progress. Sometimes I even felt guilty about recovering so quickly, when others (not receiving HBOT) still struggled. From piecing together records, I realized that I was finished with my work at the Rehabilitation Institute after only three weeks of HBOT. Dr. Katz later said he had never seen anyone with an organic brain injury recover so fast, and he dismissed me because the Rehabilitation Institute had no further services to offer!

One day, Dr. Harch came to the site of the outdoor balancing activities and insisted that I go up to the balance beams suspended thirty feet above the ground. My heart went into my throat, but he assured me that I'd be wearing safety harnesses—and a safety helmet—in case I did lose my balance. Dr. Harch brought a video camera and filmed the session, including my dramatic exit from the suspended beams when I flew down to the ground via the escape line.

It's always felt as if Dr. Harch gave me back my brain. In fact, the last SPECT brain scan indicated a near total recovery. Dr. Harch later explained that this final scan was to confirm with an image what we saw clinically. He was well pleased with the results of the treatments, and I was overjoyed.

In truth, I probably was a bit too enthusiastic about my recovery. I made plans to write a book and go on tour; specifically to address young people about avoiding the dangers and pitfalls of drug and alcohol abuse. I wanted to preach about the brain damage that could result from these substances, knowing that I could talk about what it's like to have brain damage. I was pretty passionate about the prospect of such a crusade. Later, Dr. Harch told me he had worried that he had given me too much oxygen and induced this hyperactivity.

From my perspective, in the course of five months I had been to the lowest depths of depression and then brought back to life. My mind was back, along with normal movement and an ability to make my way in the world. At the time, very few people had experienced such a recovery from brain injury with HBOT.

In late October, Mom and her friend, Pat, flew to New Orleans to meet with Dr. Harch and bring me back home. By that time, several divers staying at the La Quinta Inn while undergoing HBOT were approached by a legal team in order pursue litigation for their injuries. The lawyers approached me as well, believing that I had a strong case for a successful litigation against someone. I was clueless, since I'd always maintained that my decompression illness resulted from my own stubbornness and stupidity. Nevertheless, arrangements were made for me to meet with lawyers at a major law firm in Houston, Texas, a few days later.

It was great to see Mom after so long. Although we'd spoken often on the phone, seeing her in person was much better. This was a heartwarming reunion, made even better because my mother hadn't met Dr. Harch yet, and she was excited to meet the man she believed saved my life. In fact, the whole family still believes he is responsible for my full recovery. Had there never been a Dr. Harch, I feel certain I would have sealed my own fate with a self-inflicted gunshot wound to the head. I was so glad that my family had encouraged me to not give up five minutes before the miracle. Although it had been a very long five minutes, the miracle had happened.

Mom met Rod and Mitch at the hotel, and then I took Mom and Pat to visit Jana and Wanda at the hyperbaric unit. Later, I introduced them to the staff at the Rehabilitation Institute. The speech/language therapist was particularly interested in meeting my mother because she had questions about my hyperactive state, but Mom told her I'd always been like that. To this day, I believe I was so animated because I was filled with joy at overcoming what had seemed like a hopeless condition.

During this time, Mom and Pat and I went off to explore some sights in

New Orleans, including a visit to the French Quarter, where we enjoyed beignets at the Café Dumond. What a delight to drink great coffee and munch on the tasty beignets, but not worry about spilling food on my clothes. Of course, everyone's clothes got a bit messy from the beignets, because their powdered sugar flew all about. We also listened to jazz and blues on Bourbon Street, and at one point, Pat and I danced in the street as a Dixieland band played. We also went to a bar, the birthplace of Al's Famous Hurricane drink. Mom, who rarely drinks alcohol, got about halfway through one of the Hurricanes before asking me to pour out the rest. It was a great day of celebration.

So, how did my story turn out so well? What allowed for the miracles of recovery?

We met Dr. Harch for lunch at Algier's Landing Restaurant, which was so exciting for Mom. He arrived with my brain scans in hand, and his brilliant, intelligent eyes were filled with good humor. This was the first time I'd seen the scans. The before, during, and after images of my brain were amazing. I simply couldn't believe what I was seeing. The "holes," as Dr. Harch called them, had filled in.

The tears in my mother's eyes were those of joy. Dr. Harch told of the need to wait until my mother asked him to take on my case, before he could even consent to providing treatments. And he thought she'd never ask. For him, my case represented another breakthrough; proof (through scans to back up my obvious changes) that delayed HBOT could bring about healing, in varying degrees, in at least some situations of brain damage.

Before I left, I saw Dr. Blotner to set up the schedule for weaning off Prozac over a period of a couple of months. And I saw Dr. Mendoza for post-treatment neuropsychological tests. This time I did better, although not 100%. Still, the contrast was so huge that I could be grateful to have my brain back. I'd finally driven that spider out for good.

The time came to leave New Orleans. I couldn't help but be apprehensive. Would I regress after I left? I think my fears were normal, though, because I remembered not being able to balance or walk or think. We traveled to Houston, where I had an uneventful visit with the lawyers. From a legal standpoint, not being a commercial diver working for a firm responsible for my safety and healthcare made my situation different from the other divers. Then, on the drive home, I concentrated on savoring all the sights and smells, knowing I'd be able to remember them now.

I stayed in Portales, where my parents lived, for a day of rest before traveling across the state to my home in Farmington. In addition to going back to work, Dr. Harch asked me to do follow-up neuropsychological testing with Drs. Curley and Yoachim, but he insisted that I not tell them about the hyperbaric treatments. Dr. Harch wanted the record of the neuropsychological battery to document additional changes. I was happy to do this, both as a favor to Dr. Harch, and because I'd become interested in intelligence and neurological process assessments.

I went back to work in early November—I was back in every way. My dreadful symptoms were gone. No slurred speech or disorientation. And I could think again. Ever since the night in the hotel when I recognized that I could think again, I realized I was out of my more than three-month stupor. As the weeks passed, I felt more improvements to my overall well-being. Dr. Harch said it could happen, and it did.

Over my Christmas break that year, I returned to New Orleans for additional HBOT. I told Dr. Harch that I felt about 95% recovered, and he said it might be possible to get to 100%. He asked me to have more treatments with an increased dosage of oxygen, but I wouldn't need new imaging or other testing. Dr. Harch wanted to find out how many treatments it would take for me to feel completely returned to normal.

I enjoyed going back to New Orleans as a well person, and the additional treatments seemed to boost my recovery that much more. By this time, I had been completely weaned from Prozac, so I had my brain back in every sense. After twelve or thirteen treatments, I told Dr. Harch I felt 100% myself. At that point, he stopped the treatments and I went back home—I was truly a miracle case.

15
KEEPING UP THE GOOD FIGHT

While I readjusted to my regular life, my father considered our options for legal recourse based on presumed mistreatment of a mental disorder. Although we had a couple of appointments with attorneys, we soon realized that those institutionalized for mental illness or even brain injuries have little recourse and their rights and interests are often inadequately protected. Taking a long view, I'm not sure I was up to reliving all the medical and legal mistakes. In the end, thanks to HBOT, I returned to my life with very few side effects or deficits.

Although we took no legal action, I did experience negative consequences because of what had happened to me over the previous months. For example, a confidentiality policy was compromised when a local school counselor, who worked part-time at Sunrise, began spreading concerns about allowing a brain damaged, suicidal and homicidal maniac to teach children! My junior high principal called Dr. Harch, who reassured him that I was not a threat to children. Even after that phone call, however, the principal and assistant principal continued to proctor my teaching. One parent removed her daughter from my classroom because of the rumors. But now, after thirty-one years of working in the public schools, my record remains clear of *any* wrongdoing of any kind with children.

Now that HBOT had given me my brain back, I wanted to do more with my life. In addition to teaching, I began playing music on the weekends, even forming my own band at one point. I also became intrigued with special education in a new way. I had always learned without complication, but my brain injury increased my empathy for students who struggled. The neuropsychological and intelligence assessments that I'd encountered along the way increased my interest in the way the brain works. How does it use language or control the fine motor skills associated with writing? How do we accurately measure cognitive abilities? Why do some students learn so easily, while so many students struggle?

My curiosity led me to a master's degree program at Eastern New Mexico University that would enable me to become an educational diagnostician. As straightforward as this seemed, I was warned that the program was rigorous and hard to get through. My background in general education was questioned, and if I'd been easily discouraged I'd have left a pre-admission interview in Portales and given up the idea of pursuing this degree. But the gatekeeper of the program had no way to know that my own months of cognitive difficulties had sparked a new passion to help children with disabilities. My dilemma involved my desire to communicate my passion for the program, while not revealing the reason it had developed.

Not long after, I heard about a job opening in Portales for a math position, which also included teaching students to use computers and facilitating groups for at-risk students, similar to the support groups I ran at my school. I had concerns about my computer experience, but I enthusiastically applied for the job and sent information about every successful educational program with which I'd been involved.

I moved to Portales, started a new job, applied for graduate school, and later became one of only three to graduate from the educational diagnostics program. I soon moved from a teaching position to using assessment instruments to determine students' cognitive and achievement abilities. While in the master's program, I'd begun to have my doubts about what constituted a specific learning disability, and I soon became active in an organization that advocated for consistent programs to determine learning disabilities. I have since retired from my job as an educational diagnostician in Portales after fourteen successful years but continue to work as an educational diagnostician in Muleshoe, Texas, and consider it my mission to help children who have special needs.

My work has been singled out for recognition over the years, something that's especially sweet considering how close I came to being "shelved," as I'd put it. I've even been honored as an outstanding chess coach for the young people in our school district. The rewards in education have always extended far beyond a paycheck, and with this book finished, my next goal may be pursuing a doctorate degree.

I've also continued my music, having written several songs. My songwriting partner, Lonnie Berry, along with friends in our musical group, Spiritual Journey, faithfully stood by my side throughout my ordeals. The goal of our group is to share the love of God everywhere we go. For myself, I prefer to sing of hope and great miracles, because my life has been one such miracle.

Over these last years, I also worked on this book. Why did it take so long? I've discovered several reasons. First, it took many years to fully come to grips with my intense emotions during the months of misdiagnosis and, in some cases, mistreatment. To this day, I've never fully made peace with the seven days of incarceration in the county jail. The psychological torture alone was more than I care to remember. However, I know in my heart that God will help me eventually come to peace.

I didn't seek help to deal with these feelings, because I didn't want to be handed a prescription for a drug to help me feel better, when I needed to work through them myself. I didn't (and still don't) trust psychological intervention very much either, and feared that through this process my mental state would deteriorate rather than improve. Of course, I continued my sobriety and worked to improve my mental health through my support group. I found that as I lived more and more in the solution, the past injustices were left behind.

I never stopped being amazed that I could return to my life, and I resolved to live it to the fullest. I traveled extensively in Europe, the United States, and Mexico, and also traveled all over northern New Mexico and southern Colorado to play with various bands. In other words, I stopped saying "someday," and instead, made the most of every day. Years passed as I was "living in the now."

During these years, I became involved in educational research and presented papers at meetings of the Council for Exceptional Children as well as at the National Council for Teaching Mathematics. I stayed involved with the head of the educational diagnostic program, Dr. Shaughnessy, and traveled with him to Scotland and Poland to present educational research.

Unfortunately, life is not a fairytale and not all endings are happy. As an educational diagnostician I have at times become disillusioned about the current state of education, or more precisely, the lack of advancement in the field. Over the years, I've quipped that it seems we dumb down the U.S. schools on purpose. Since I don't like to dwell in negativity, I continue to trudge along attempting to help special needs children as best I can.

One area that continues to trouble me involves lack of critical thinking and problem solving skills among our students. More and more, these higher levels of thought have been replaced with the lowest level of learning—memorization of trivial facts, bits and pieces here and there. I believe the United States faces a severe shortage of its greatest resource—free thinking. I could get on my bandwagon about the emptiness of mass media, and the way in which they attempt to homogenize our children. I realize that we have pockets of excellence, but I can't help but wonder from which public schools our future Dr. Harches will come. Perhaps I sound like some teachers you know. But it's possible to love teaching children and still become disillusioned with the institutions of education. On a daily basis, I find I must turn over my concerns to God.

In these intervening years, I've enjoyed the company of my immediate family and friends. I'm still in contact with my good friend Lee Ann, who remained my friend and prayer partner through my struggles. We often joke that she and her children were the subjects of many of my cognitive, achievement, and processing testing practices required in graduate school. Her three children would see me coming and say, "Oh no, here comes Dan again. I wonder what he is going to test us with now." I'm very grateful to those kids for indulging me, and for the fact that Lee Ann never gave up on me. She prayed me through my sickness, never doubting that I would be healed.

It's difficult to write about a few things. For example, some years back, just after I had completed my post graduate work to become an educational diagnostician, I met someone and remarried, but things went badly and we divorced after two years. Ironically, the painful divorce forced me to relive the nightmare of my illness. There is no need to go into great detail, but let's just say that during our divorce proceedings my soon-to-be former wife took selected portions of my medical records to share with my school superintendent in an attempt to discredit me and have me dismissed from my job. None of what she took included my correct diagnosis nor the records of my recovery.

This was a devastating blow, and I nearly quit my job over the whole incident. It eventually resolved, with Dr. Harch once again stepping in to verify that I was not dangerous to children and was capable of doing my job. Fortunately, my immediate supervisor believed in me and my dedication to helping children with exceptionalities. Unfortunately, we had quite a go round over this bitter divorce. I was completely shocked by how bad it became. Letters went back and forth between my supervisor and Dr. Harch, who had to explain that my former wife had taken my father's notes that documented my pre-HBOT struggles. I feared reprisals at school, even from my colleagues, once this information circulated, but in the end my now ex-wife's actions were seen as a vicious attempt to destroy me.

In order to continue my sobriety, my spiritual program requires me to forgive and avoid harboring resentments, and eventually I came to forgive my ex-wife. As for Dr. Clairemont, the man who sent me from the hospital to the jail in handcuffs, I never kept up with him, but one day I learned that he had died from a self-inflicted gunshot wound. News of Dr. Clairemont's death spread quickly through the mental health community, and for me, it again raised questions about what happens to the most vulnerable patients.

I often think back to the people I met in the mental hospitals, many of whom were not spared the fate of lifelong institutionalization. One young man, an Elvis wannabe, shared his story of singing in a local band in the northern mountains of New Mexico. Everything in his life was humming along nicely until he had a serious car accident. No one could have known by looking at him how extensively he suffered. His life became a series of jail cells and mental wards, leading him to compare one place to another and give his opinions about which hospital had better drugs. So many years later, I reflect about this young man and the tragedy of his life, especially the brain damage from his accident. Could Dr. Harch have helped him? I'll never know for sure, but I believe he, too, might have been given his brain back. Dr. Harch has treated patients like this man and he's told me stories about their recovery.

I think about Marcia, who had warned me about botching a suicide and ending up in a persistent vegetative state, and wonder what happened to her. I can't forget the man from Gallup, New Mexico, whose son and daughter-in-law were killed by a drunk driver. Earlier I wrote about the violent acts he committed against people he saw leaving bars and getting into their cars. In his mind, he would stop at nothing to prevent impaired individuals from endangering others. Did he ever let go of his anger and resentment? I don't know and probably never will.

Just in those few months, I met so many people whose lives had taken such tragic turns, often as a result of a brain injury. In some cases, these individuals had nothing visibly wrong with them, but they were damaged all the same. Maybe one day, they will receive HBOT as a matter of course, because in the future I have no doubt it will be accepted as a viable treatment for brain injuries, visible or not. It may not bring everyone back 100%, but I know it rescues many. As I sit in the comfort of a rescued life, a life redeemed from great tragedy, I wonder what became of these men and women.

I've also come to terms with various members of my family, who even now don't understand the full measure of what happened to me. Some still hold on to the belief that I suffered a psychological disorder. But the ordeal actually gave me something precious, a wonderful relationship with my father. He never gave up on me; he pursued every possible avenue to save my life. Of course, my mother and brother were there by his side as well. I know that I wouldn't be alive today had it not been for my immediate family.

While in graduate school, I wrote a paper on thrill-seeking and the kind of personality that drives people to crave the extra stimulation that most ordinary people don't need. I am confident that I was one such person, but I have since happily discarded that label. Every now and then I'll joke about taking up sky diving or some other daring pursuit, but I know I'll leave those things to others. My recovery allowed me to do valuable things, and I don't seek such extreme thrills any longer.

One reason I wrote this book is to be of help to others. Today, the news is filled with stories of brain injured soldiers returning from our two wars. Dr. Harch has been able to treat some of our young veterans with traumatic brain injury (TBI), and is consistently showing positive results. Currently, he's working to see that HBOT is offered routinely to brain-injured veterans. It is my dream that the families of these soldiers will read my story and find new hope in the possibilities of recovery. I also hope these families—and all citizens—will fight to get our returning military men and women the help they need. I realize that the military rehabilitation facilities are superior in quality and many miracles occur in them. However, if one important treatment isn't available, then recovery may be compromised—it's less than it could be.

Dr. Harch has reminded me that by the time I came to New Orleans I'd been seen by over *twenty* different doctors, psychiatrists, and psychologists. While in New Orleans, I saw many more, eventually reaching a total of thirty-five. No wonder I sometimes questioned the cause of my illness or became tempted to believe that nothing could be done for me. I know that thousands, perhaps millions of people are making the same kind of rounds, going from doctor to doctor looking for help. How remarkable that they keep searching, keep fighting. So many families are like mine; they simply refuse to give up. At one point, a psychiatrist turned to my mother and said, "Mrs. Greathouse, you can take your son to all the doctors in the world, but he will never be well. You can even take him to some quack in New Orleans, but you will be wasting your money."

Needless to say, I'm incredibly grateful that my parents did not listen to that so-called expert. Fortunately, some professionals are willing to look past the easy explanations that lead to truncated searches and quick solutions based on limited information. These professionals helped fuel my passion for educational diagnostics and avoiding the mistakes that slap labels onto children too quickly. I was once a "problem patient," just as so many young children are "problem students."

In thinking about what happened to me, I realize that I've written this book to give a voice to those who don't fit into easy diagnostic categories— challenging students, brain-injured patients, wounded veterans, and all who could be helped if we cast aside old assumptions and quit settling for second best.

The first day I met Dr. Harch, I pled, *"Doc, I want my brain back."*

Against all odds and all of the scoffing naysayers' doubts, Dr. Harch gave me back my brain, and now I want to help others experience the same miracle.

AUTHOR'S NOTE

So many wonderful things have happened since my successful treatment twenty-two years ago. Russell Ouart, one of the veterans who were successfully treated with Dr. Harch's hyperbaric oxygen therapy protocol for traumatic brain injury/posttraumatic stress disorder, and whom I met at a fundraiser in New York State on Veteran's Day in 2009, has finally received the Purple Heart.

John Salcedo, from LA City Films, a very artistic and passionate filmmaker, whom I also first met on Veteran's Day in 2009, continues to produce *Brain Storm* academic films documenting the evolution of hyperbaric medicine research by Paul G. Harch, MD at LSU School of Medicine to calm the storm inside the brain of the brain injured.

I contacted John on July 13, 2013, to enlist him for further filming during a trip to New Orleans twenty-two years after my successful treatment for chronic brain injury. Salcedo filmed interviews with several current patients, Dr. Harch, and me, along with footage of the actual road trip retracing my original journey from New Mexico to New Orleans. Some of the resulting footage has been edited into *Brain Storm: "Break the Silence"* which begs the viewer to question why one of the most revolutionary brain repair therapies ever to be discovered and verified in the history of medicine is not recognized or utilized by the VA to rescue at-risk veterans from suicide. Why does the FDA not recognize this therapy? Why have the top levels of the Pentagon refused to utilize this protocol to save veterans suffering from TBI and PTSD? What about the possibilities for the thousands of individuals who suffer from brain injuries each year? When, in God's name, will the silence be broken? Just as the Constant Halo song begs, we beg for divine intervention to break this incredible and inexplicable silence, because the powers that be have turned a deaf ear to all of the suffering souls.

Meanwhile, Dr. Harch, without FDA approval, without VA approval, and without being sanctioned by medical insurance, diligently continues his work, helping to restore lives just as he did mine twenty-two years ago.

ADDITIONAL RESOURCES

The Oxygen Revolution, Paul Harch, MD, and Virginia McCullough (Hatherleigh Press 2007)

HBOT Online, www.HBOT.com This website includes information contributed by Dr. Harch and offers links to other sources, or call toll free 855-GET-HBOT (855-438-4268)

Consultations with Dr. Harch are welcome and encouraged:

Dr. Paul G. Harch, or
Juliette Lucarani
Harch Hyperbarics Inc.
5216 Lapalco Blvd
Marrero, LA 70072
(504) 309-4948

The reader may wish to help stop the veteran suicides that are occurring each day by sending donations to:

The Greater New Orleans Foundation
1055 St. Charles Ave, Suite 100
New Orleans, LA 70130

Write on the memo line: For the Harch Hyperbaric Research Fund

Or donate online at www.GNOF.org, click the large green "Give" button and follow the instructions. Again, designate the donation for: The Harch Hyperbaric Research Fund.

APPENDIX

The Basics of Hyperbaric Oxygen Therapy

Although I urge you to read Dr. Harch's book, *The Oxygen Revolution*, I also want to provide some basic information about the treatment here. In short, hyperbaric oxygen therapy, known as HBOT, harnesses the power of *oxygen under pressure*, and it has the ability to act on every cell in the body. In fact, HBOT acts like a drug, in that it affects the DNA of each cell. Multiple HBO treatments (usually about twenty-five to thirty) stimulates the DNA in each cell and results in permanent rejuvenation of damaged cells. In other words, applying hyperbaric oxygen to the cells is not just a superficial remedy that acts on symptoms, but rather, attempts to repair the damaged cells and return their function.

HBOT acts on tissues that have been deprived of oxygen. At one time, it was thought that a damaged cell could not be repaired or "revived." (Some medical professionals still believe that damaged neurons, brain cells, cannot be altered.) However, over the years, HBOT has been shown to have a beneficial effect on every cell in the body, including neurons. Dr. Harch and others demonstrate the changes in the brain brought about by HBOT through SPECT scans, which I referred to in the book. Changes in the brain also are evident because of drastic improvements in patients like me.

In my case, a diving accident damaged my brain; in others, a stroke or a neurological disease, such as Alzheimer's or multiple sclerosis has deprived the tissues of oxygen. HBOT also is used for wound healing—diabetic foot wounds, for example, and birth injuries resulting in brain damage (cerebral palsy), bone infections, and burns. The list of applications continues to grow, and some practitioners have used HBOT for conditions such as autism, alcohol detoxification, anti-aging/rejuvenation, and medical emergencies such as carbon monoxide poisoning and incidents of near drowning.

HBOT is used in both acute situations, such as following a diving accident, and in chronic diseases, such as months or years after an injury. That's what happened to me; my success (and of thousands of others) goes to illustrate the promise of helping millions of individuals recover to at least some degree from traumatic brain injury (TBI). This includes those whose brain injuries resulted from accidents, of course, but it also addresses the many thousands of soldiers who have sustained TBI in our current wars.

More HBOT clinics exist today than were available when I received treatment in the 1990s. Although some patients must plan a three week (or more) stay in lodging near the clinic, many more are able to find treatment facilities closer to home. Treatments for chronic conditions, i.e., delayed treatment for TBI, diabetic foot wounds, and so forth, are delivered in what is known as *blocks*, usually 40 or so. On the other hand, treatment for acute conditions, such as near-drowning or carbon monoxide poisoning, require only a few treatments—delivered early—to stop the inflammatory process that occurs at the time of an injury.

The use of HBOT for both acute and chronic conditions makes it especially important to investigate facilities in your area. Take the time to learn if your local hospitals currently have hyperbaric chambers and for what conditions they use them. I also urge you to make use of the resources listed in this book to further educate yourself about this very special treatment that holds so much promise for human well-being.

ABOUT THE AUTHOR

Doc, I Want My Brain Back is the compelling true story about a scuba diver who suffered a brain injury and was misdiagnosed by well over thirty medical professionals before receiving successful treatment. After being jailed and committed to the state mental hospital, the diver's parents intervened and made provisions for him to be transferred to another mental hospital, where he was improperly drugged with pharmaceutical psychotropic medications.

Meanwhile, most of his friends and family "wrote him off" as merely another mental case; however, his father researched delayed hyperbaric oxygen treatments, well outside of the prescribed limitations and found supporting evidence for a therapy that Dr. Paul G. Harch had successfully applied to another diver.

Unlike any other brain injury rehabilitation book, *Doc, I Want My Brain Back* chronicles the events of Dan Greathouse's life that led Dr. Harch to discover the tip of the iceberg for neurorehabilitation. With this successful case in brain injury repair, Hyperbaric oxygen therapy takes its place in medical history. *Doc, I Want My Brain Back* is the story of a medical breakthrough written from the patient's perspective.

Visit Dan at dangreathouse.com for more details on his books and to read his blog.